Mental Health Issues
of Child Maltreatment

Contemporary Strategies

Volume 1: Presentation and Assessment

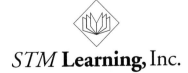

STM **Learning,** Inc.

Leading Publisher of Scientific, Technical, and Medical Educational Resources
Saint Louis
www.stmlearning.com

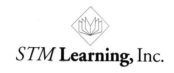

STM Learning, Inc.

We've partnered with Copyright Clearance Center to make it easy for you to request permissions to reuse content from STM Learning, Inc.

With copyright.com, you can quickly and easily secure the permissions you want.

Simply follow these steps to get started:

— Visit **copyright.com** and enter the title, ISBN, or ISSN number of the publication you'd like to reuse and hit "Go."
— After finding the title you'd like, choose "Pay-Per-Use Options."
— Enter the publication year of the content you'd like to reuse.
— Scroll down the list to find the type of reuse you want to request.
— Select the corresponding bubble and click "Price & Order."
— Fill out any required information and follow the prompts to acquire the proper permissions to reuse the content that you'd like.

For questions about using the service on **copyright.com**, please contact:

Copyright Clearance Center
222 Rosewood Drive
Danvers, MA 01923
Phone: +1-(978) 750-8400
Fax: +1-(978) 750-4470

Additional requests can be sent directly to **info@copyright.com**.

Mental Health Issues
of Child Maltreatment

Contemporary Strategies
Volume 1: Presentation and Assessment

Paul Thomas Clements, PhD, RN, ANEF, DF-IAFN, DF-AFN
Clinical Professor
Center for Excellence in Forensic Nursing
Texas A&M University
College Station, TX
President-Elect
Academy of Forensic Nursing

David T. Solomon, PhD, HSP-P
Associate Professor/Director of Health Services Psychology
PsyD Program
Department of Psychology
Western Carolina University
Cullowhee, NC

Beth I. Barol, PhD, LSW, BCB, NADD-CC
Associate Dean (Retired)
Widener University Center for Social Work Education
Consultant (National and International)
Institute Director
Pennsylvania Capacity Building Institute
Ridley Park, PA

Ciera E. Schoonover, PhD, MSW, MPH, HSP
Assistant Professor
Department of Psychology
Middle Tennessee State University
Murfreesboro, TN

Soraya Seedat, PhD, MBChB, FC Psych (SA), MMed Psych, MPhil Applied Ethics (Bioethics)
Distinguished Professor and Executive Head
Department of Psychiatry
Stellenbosch University
Cape Town, South Africa

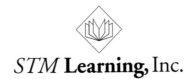

STM **Learning,** Inc.

Leading Publisher of Scientific, Technical, and Medical Educational Resources
Saint Louis
www.stmlearning.com

Publishers: Glenn E. Whaley and Marianne V. Whaley
Managing Editor: Samantha Brown
Graphic Design Director: Glenn E. Whaley
Graphic Designer: Connie H. C. Wang
Curriculum Developer: Samantha Brown
Associate Editors: Miya Russell, Tammy Arnow, Gracie York
Copy Editors: Miya Russell, Katie Slaten
Proofreaders: Katie Slaten, Tammy Arnow, Gracie York

Printed in the United States of America.

Publisher:
STM Learning, Inc.
Saint Louis, Missouri 63033
Phone: (314) 434-2424
http://www.stmlearning.com orders@stmlearning.com

Print ISBN: 9781953119209
eBook ISBN: 9781953119216

Library of Congress Cataloging-in-Publication Data

Names: Clements, Paul T. (Paul Thomas), 1962- editor. | Solomon, David T.,
    editor. | Schoonover, Ciera, editor. | Barol, Beth I., editor. | Seedat,
    Soraya, 1966- editor.
Title: Mental health issues of child maltreatment : contemporary strategies
    / [edited by] Paul Thomas Clements, David T. Solomon, Ciera Schoonover,
    Beth I. Barol, Soraya Seedat.
Description: Saint Louis : STM Learning, Inc., [2023]- | Includes
    bibliographical references. | Contents: v. 1. Presentations & assessment
    | Summary: "A contemporary overview of strategies to identify and assess
    mental health issues arising from child maltreatment"-- Provided by
    publisher.
Identifiers: LCCN 2023046741 | ISBN 9781953119209 (v. 1 ; paperback) | ISBN
    9781953119216 (v. 1 ; ebook)
Subjects: MESH: Child Abuse--psychology | Stress Disorders,
    Traumatic--diagnosis | Adverse Childhood Experiences | Child
Classification: LCC RC569.5.C55 | NLM WS 350.8.A2 | DDC
    616.85/82230019--dc23/eng/20231113
LC record available at https://lccn.loc.gov/2023046741

Contributors

Hela Baer, LCSW, E-RYT
Licensed Clinical Social Worker/Experienced Registered
Yoga teacher/Equine Specialist
Alexandria Place Therapy
Alexandria, VA

Alexandra L. Ballinger, MA
Doctoral Student, Clinical Science
Department of Psychology
Michigan State University
East Lansing, MI

Beth I. Barol, PhD, LSW, BCB, NADD-CC
Associate Dean (Retired)
Widener University Center for Social Work Education
Consultant (national and international)
Institute Director
Pennsylvania Capacity Building Institute
Ridley Park, PA

Jacob R. Brown, BS
Graduate Research Assistant
Department of Psychological Sciences
Kent State University
Kent, OH

Sarah H. Buffie, MSW, LSW
Founder/Director/Lead Trainer/Consultant
Soul Bird Consulting
Cincinnati, OH

Brian Cheline, MA
Ball State University

Paul Thomas Clements, PhD, RN, ANEF, DF-IAFN, DF-AFN
Clinical Professor
Center for Excellence in Forensic Nursing
Texas A&M University
College Station, TX
President-Elect
Academy of Forensic Nursing

Andrew Davis, PhD
Head of the School of Education/Associate Dean
College of Community Engagement and Professions
University of Wisconsin-Milwaukee
Milwaukee, WI

Rachel S. Faulkenberry, BS
Department of Psychology
Western Carolina University
Cullowhee, NC

Theresa Fay-Hillier, DrPH, MSN, PMHCNS-BC
Associate Clinical Professor
College of Nursing and Health Professions
Drexel University
Philadelphia, PA

Lia Field Martin, PhD
Associate Director of Quality Management
Justice Resource Institute
Needham, MA

Mitzy D. Flores, PhDc, MSN, RN, AHN-BC, CHSE, COI, Caritas Coach©, Introspective Hypnosis Practitioner
Visiting Professor/Academic and Clinical Nurse Educator
School of Nursing
University of South Florida
Tampa, FL

Adam D. Hicks, MA
Doctoral Intern
Department of Psychology
Western Carolina University
Cullowhee, NC

Tami L. Jakubowski, DNP, CPNP-PC, CSN
Associate Professor
Department of Nursing
The College of New Jersey
Ewing, NJ

Sara Jones, PhD, APRN, PMHNP-BC, FAAN, FAANP
Associate Professor
College of Nursing and Health Professions
McNeese State University
Lake Charles, LA
Owner/APRN
Journey Wellness Clinic
North Little Rock, AR

Stevie B. Knight, MA
Ball State University

Alytia Levendosky, PhD
Professor/Director of Clinical Training
Department of Psychology
Michigan State University
East Lansing, MI

David M. McCord, PhD
Emeritus Professor of Clinical Psychology
Department of Psychology
Western Carolina University
Cullowhee, NC

Tania E. Morales Zelaya, MA
Ball State University

Clariana Vitória Ramos de Oliveira, PhD, MSc, RN
Assistant Professor
School of Nursing
University of Nevada, Las Vegas
Las Vegas, NV

Caitlin Rancher, PhD
Postdoctoral Fellow
Department of Psychiatry & Behavioral Sciences
Medical University of South Carolina
Charleston, SC

Megan E. Slagel, MA
Doctoral Candidate
Department of Educational Psychology
Ball State University
Muncie, IN

Daniel W. Smith, PhD
Professor
Department of Psychiatry and Behavioral Sciences
Medical University of South Carolina
Charleston, SC

David T. Solomon, PhD, HSP-P
Associate Professor/ Director of Health Services Psychology
PsyD Program
Department of Psychology
Western Carolina University
Cullowhee, NC

FOREWORD

In 1988, I was a newly minted prosecutor working in a rural county of approximately 13 000 people. As is often the case with new prosecutors, I was assigned to handle the less glamorous cases that rarely catch the public's eye—child protection cases, juvenile justice cases, and criminal cases involving interpersonal violence in which children were witnesses to the cruelties adults inflict on one another.

If truth be told, none of us back then knew what we were doing—not the judges, prosecutors, defense attorneys, child protection workers, law enforcement officers, medical or mental health professionals. This was approximately a decade before the publication of "Adverse Childhood Experience"[1] research and terms such as "poly-victimization"[2] and "trauma-informed practice"[3] were not yet in our vocabulary.

We were not far removed from high-profile daycare cases in which well-intentioned professionals unaware of child development, linguistics, and other factors that need to be considered when interviewing young children, made errors which resulted in the overturning of convictions. The collection of evidence was also very different back then. Cell phones, the internet, laptops, and other technology were not widely used.

We have come a long way since then. Today, there are over 950 Children's Advocacy Centers serving nearly every community in the United States. We now implement forensic interview training programs to thousands of frontline interviewers as well as other members of the medical community.[4] The growth of the internet and cell phone usage made it easier to locate and sexually abuse children, but it also created an online footprint that makes it easier to prosecute those who prey on children. Although still in its infancy, there is even movement to develop spiritual care workers or specially trained chaplains who can respond to the spiritual impact of child abuse.[5]

Perhaps the most exciting development in recent decades is the idea that the past need not be prologue and that, working together, we can significantly reduce child abuse.

There is a simple reason for the decline in child abuse: we have dramatically improved the education of teachers, doctors, nurses, child protection workers, criminal justice professionals and medical and mental health providers to prevent abuse and, when it cannot be prevented, to respond with excellence.

This is why the publication of *Mental Health Issues of Child Maltreatment* is so important. In these pages, frontline professionals of today and tomorrow will find concrete, research-supported responses to nearly every aspect of child maltreatment. Perhaps best viewed as a toolkit, this invaluable resource will guide these professionals to even greater heights of responding to child maltreatment in a trauma-informed manner.

Although the complete eradication of child abuse may not be within our grasp anytime soon, it is clear we are making great strides, and the best is yet to come. To that end, *Mental Health Issues of Child Maltreatment* is a welcome addition to the child protection canon.

Victor I. Vieth, JD[6]
Director, Center for Faith & Child Protection

REFERENCES

1. Vincent Felitti & Robert F. Anda, *The Relationship of Adverse Childhood Experiences to Adult Medical Disease, Psychiatric Disorders and Sexual Behavior: Implications for Healthcare,* in Ruthe A. Lanius, eric Vermeten & Clare Pain (EDS) The Impact of Early Life Trauma on Health and Disease: The Hidden Epidemic 77 (Cambridge Medicine 2010).

2. Heather A. Turner, David Finkelhor, and Richard Ormrod, *Poly-Victimization in a National Sample of Children and Youth,* 38(3) American Journal of Preventive Medicine 323 (2010), David Finkelhor, Richard K. Omrod, Heather A. Turner, *Poly-victimization: A Neglected Component in Child Victimization,* 31 Journal of Child Abuse & Neglect 7 (2007).

3. SAMHSA's Concept of Trauma and Guidance for a Trauma-Informed Approach. HHS Publication No. (SMA) 14-4884. Rockville, MD: Substance Abuse and Mental Health Services Administration, 2014.

4. Rita Farrell and Victor Vieth, *ChildFirst® forensic interview training program,* 32(2) APSAC Advisor 56-63 (2020); Kathleen Coulborn Faller, *Forty Years of Forensic Interviewing of Children Suspected of Sexual Abuse, 1974-2014: Historical Benchmarks,* 4 Social Sciences 34, 49 (2015).

5. Victor I. Vieth, Mark D. Everson, Viola Vaughan-Eden, Suzanna Tiapula, Shauna Galloway-Williams, Carrie Nettles, *Keeping Faith: The Potential Role of a Chaplain to Address the Spiritual Needs of Maltreated Children and Advise Child Abuse Multi-Discplinary Teams,* 14(2) Liberty University Law Review 351 (2020).

6. Chief Program Officer for Education & Research, Zero Abuse Project. Mr. Vieth is a former child abuse prosecutor who received national attention for his work to address child abuse in rural communities. He went on to direct the National Center for Prosecution of Child Abuse. He is the recipient of the Victim Rights Legend Award from the United States Department of Justice, the Lifetime Achievement Award from the Institute on Violence, Abuse & Trauma (IVAT), and the Change Maker Award from the Academy on Violence & Abuse.

Preface

Within the idealized social construct of "childhood," what comes to mind is images of laughter, joy, and play; however, for many children, the reality is a developmental timeline filled with Adverse Childhood Experiences (ACEs)[1] that threaten physical safety and emotional wellbeing. Child maltreatment is a global public health concern, spanning all social classes, cultures, economic contexts, and ethnicities. Children represent the very future of our existence and require careful nurturing from the adults in their lives. However, oftentimes, those entrusted with the most care—parents—are the primary perpetrators of abuse. Offenders can also include other family members, teachers, friends, coaches, neighbors, medical professionals, and spiritual advisors. Child maltreatment often co-occurs with other forms of victimization, such as witnessing family or community violence, cybercrimes, and more. In this book, the authors advocate a trauma-informed approach to care, beginning with understanding that the complexities of childhood trauma can result from a single event, series of events, or set of circumstances. The circumstances can be experienced physically or emotionally, from a harmful or life-threatening event (real or perceived). The resulting trauma has lasting adverse effects on the child or family functioning, and mental, physical, social, emotional, or spiritual wellbeing.[2,3] As the scope of professionals studying childhood maltreatment and trauma continues to expand, so has our understanding of the wide-reaching effects and manifestations of abuse.

Child maltreatment has long-lasting deleterious effects on brain development, with its rapidly scaffolding architecture, and delicate circuitry-associated functioning. Child maltreatment also affects immune function, endocrine regulation, and metabolic health.[4] The diminished sense of self that often results from child maltreatment can increase the risk of mental illness, substance misuse, suicidality, learning problems, social problems with other children and adults, teen pregnancy, lack of success in school, interpersonal violence, and chronic illness.[5] Risk of maladaptive functioning can be significant during childhood, but problems can also persist into adulthood. Despite these grave physical and mental health consequences, the vast majority of child victims never seek or receive help due to a wide variety of challenging social determinants of health that interfere with or prevent access to care. Many do not have the social context to realize that their experience of maltreatment is out of the ordinary and worthy of support for recovery.[6,7] Additionally, children who grow up experiencing violence are at risk of re-enacting it as young adults and caregivers themselves, creating a new generation of victims.[8]

Fortunately, as professionals or concerned adults, we can do quite a bit for children who are at risk of, or who are currently, experiencing child abuse. Learning more about child abuse is an important first step. Early intervention can disrupt the cycle of violence and re-traumatization. The authors within this book present strategies for assessment as well as multifaceted and concurrent interventions responding to how children's traumatic reactions to violence, neglect, and abuse may be influenced by their individual characteristics and developmental factors. Children suffering from violence and neglect are often powerless and have been called "invisible victims" of interpersonal and intimate partner violence in order to highlight their position on the periphery of what has traditionally been seen as an adult problem. Sometimes, a child's silence can be mistaken for resilience, leading to missed opportunities for therapeutic intervention. Though adults might wish their conflicts occurred in a vacuum, children often see, hear, and react to situations of domestic violence even more than their caregivers would believe. The myth of children sleeping through violent incidents during the night or having no knowledge of the abuse occurring in the home needs to be confronted and dispelled. Down the road, exposure to domestic violence early in life increases the risk of girls becoming victimized as they grow up and boys becoming perpetrators of violence later in life. This book aims to help professionals disrupt that cycle of invisibility, missed interventions, and lifelong aftershocks.

The authors propose that there is no microcosmic solution to any childhood event; rather, that all trauma-informed approaches are geared toward discovering strategies and identifying tools that empower children and their families for adaptively healing from their trauma and safely engaging in daily living. This will require establishing connections at the community and systems levels via referral and interdisciplinary collaboration. To reflect this need, the authors have made the conscious decision for this book to move away from a silo-based approach and toward one that reaches across disciplines and increases and enhances multi-modal communication and collaboration.

Ultimately, this is a book for the professional in need of a quick, yet evidence-based, resource check, and a source for the student who is just learning about the scope of child maltreatment. It is not limited to a particular discipline or part of the globe. Specifically, in direct response to the overarching and overwhelming needs of this vulnerable population of at-risk children, *Mental Health Issues of Child Maltreatment* intends to do the following:

— **Define the problem** of child maltreatment conceptually and numerically, using statistics that describe the state of maltreatment and the characteristics of those most affected by it

— **Identify causes and risk factors** that appear to affect susceptibility to maltreatment, such as factors that increase a child's risk of abuse or obstacles to delivering effective child protection services

— **Design interventions** that are trauma-informed, sensitive, and developmentally targeted for children and their caregivers

— **Disseminate information** about the evidence and effectiveness of these interventions to increase the profile for their usage in clinical practice

— **Educate students and future professionals** in psychology, medicine, nursing, social work, and creative arts therapies to mitigate the effects of child maltreatment for future generations

It is with these thoughts and intentions that we, both individually and collectively, are hopeful that the following chapters will provide support and guidance to you, the reader, in your efforts toward providing trauma-informed care to children seeking mental health care during a time or times of need. The world, indeed, can be a complex and often traumatic place for children to navigate. We are optimistic that the information contained within this book can provide direction during the journey.

Paul Thomas Clements, PhD, RN, ANEF, DF-IAFN, DF-AFN

David T. Solomon, PhD, HSP-P

Beth I. Barol, PhD, LSW, BCB, NADD-CC

Ciera E. Schoonover, PhD, MSW, MPH, HSP

Soraya Seedat, PhD, MBChB, FC Psych (SA), MMed Psych, MPhil Applied Ethics (Bioethics)

REFERENCES

1. About the CDC-Kaiser ACE study. Centers for Disease Control and Prevention. Updated April 6, 2021. https://www.cdc.gov/violenceprevention/aces/about.html

2. SAMHSA's Trauma and Justice Strategic Initiative. SAMHSA's concept of trauma and guidance for a trauma-informed approach. 2014. https://store.samhsa.gov/sites/default/files/sma14-4884.pdf

3. *Diagnostic and Statistical Manual of Mental Disorders.* 5th ed, text rev. American Psychiatric Association. 2022. https://doi.org/10.1176/appi.books.9780890425787

4. Child Welfare Information Gateway. Child maltreatment and brain development: a primer for child welfare professionals. US Department of Health and Human Services; 2023. https://cwig-prod-prod-drupal-s3fs-us-east-1.s3.amazonaws.com/public/documents/brain_development.pdf?VersionId=C5CWzPNoORYpMKDl8YPWO6GDqi28Qh6I

5. Child maltreatment. World Health Organization. September 19, 2022. https://www.who.int/news-room/fact-sheets/detail/child-maltreatment

6. Healthy people 2030. US Department of Health and Human Services. 2023. https://health.gov/healthypeople/priority-areas

7. Reinert M, Fritze D, Nguyen T. The state of mental health in America 2023. Mental Health America; October 2022. https://mhanational.org/sites/default/files/2023-State-of-Mental-Health-in-America-Report.pdf

8. Understanding child trauma. Substance Abuse and Mental Health Administration. Updated March 17, 2023. https://www.samhsa.gov/child-trauma/understanding-child-trauma

Our Mission

To become the world leader in publishing and

information services on child abuse,

maltreatment, diseases, and domestic violence.

We seek to heighten awareness of these issues

and provide relevant information to

professionals and consumers.

Reviews

The authors have expertly woven together a comprehensive exploration of children who have encountered Adverse Childhood Experiences that is both informative and engaging. This book is an indispensable resource for anyone in the field of child maltreatment, offering a wealth of knowledge, practical guidance, and insightful perspectives.

The authors' deep understanding of forensic issues is evident throughout the book, making it a trusted companion for professionals, students, and anyone interested in the subject. The content is well-structured and covers a wide range of essential topics, from evidence collection and documentation to legal considerations and the emotional aspects of patient care.

One of the book's notable strengths is its commitment to staying current with the latest advancements and best practices in forensic mental health. It not only provides a solid foundation but also incorporates up-to-date information and case studies, ensuring that readers are well prepared to meet the challenges of this dynamic field.

What sets Mental Health Issues of Child Maltreatment *apart is its compassionate approach. The authors pay special attention to the emotional and psychological needs of patients, which is a critical aspect of our work. This focus on holistic care makes it an invaluable resource for anyone striving to excel in the field of child maltreatment.*

Overall, the authors have crafted a must-read book that combines expertise with empathy, making it an indispensable reference for mental health professionals and an enlightening read for anyone interested in this essential field of health care. I wholeheartedly recommend Mental Health Issues of Child Maltreatment *to all those committed to providing the highest standard of care and justice.*

Ann Wolbert Burgess
Professor
William Connell School of Nursing
Boston College
Chestnut Hill, MA

Mental Health Issues of Child Maltreatment *is a long overdue comprehensive resource that should be required reading for all mental health professionals, child welfare workers, court personnel and administrators—in fact, all who come into contact with survivors of child maltreatment. The text addresses the biological and neurological manifestations and consequences of child maltreatment, providing an up-to-date review of the state-of-the-art of our understanding of the sequelae of trauma. The text goes on to provide a thorough review of the challenges of accurate assessment and offers the reader a number of innovative strategies for effective interventions. Finally, the reader is presented with the challenges and strategies for extending our understanding in these areas through research. In summary, this text is an important contribution to capturing what we currently know about child maltreatment and trauma and how to intervene appropriately and effectively.*

Paula Silver, PhD
Educator and Administrator
Retired Dean
School of Human Services
Widener University
Chester, PA

This two-volume book offers a fresh perspective of childhood trauma for multidisciplinary professionals. It both questions past methods and offers successful approaches to thinking about, assessing, and treating children. The book has thoughtful, practical, and clinically relevant material for thinking about children who are now adults. Children are our future, and this book promotes means to prevent childhood maltreatment and promote their wellbeing. It honors what a whole person and whole family may need. The books highlight that children do not know what to ask for when they have had adverse childhood experiences. They do not have the resources to work on understanding and influencing what has happened to them. It is clearly up to clinical practitioners to recognize and treat the whole person, a whole family, and overarching systems.

I highly recommend this two-volume book, as it is comprehensive, clear, and compassionate in assessing and treating these often "invisible victims."

Ginny Focht-New, PhD, PMH-CNS, BCB, NADD-CC, BCN

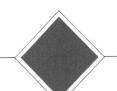

Contents in Brief

CONTENTS IN DETAIL

Mental Health Issues
of Child Maltreatment

Contemporary Strategies

Volume 1: Presentation and Assessment

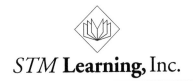

STM **Learning,** Inc.

Leading Publisher of Scientific, Technical, and Medical Educational Resources
Saint Louis
www.stmlearning.com

I

Biology and Presentation of Trauma

Child Abuse and The Emergence of Developmental Trauma

Hela Baer, LCSW, E-RYT

Objectives

After reading this chapter, the reader will be able to:

1. *Define developmental trauma and how it differs from single incident trauma.*

2. *Describe the primary symptom categories for the proposed Developmental Trauma Disorder (DTD) diagnosis and the existing Post-Traumatic Stress Disorder (PTSD) diagnosis.*

3. *Identify prominent approaches to treating developmental trauma.*

Background and Significance

Nearly 1/2 of all children in the United States have experienced at least 1 traumatic event before the age of 17 years,[1] and at least 1 in 7 children will have been exposed to developmental trauma, such as maltreatment, abuse, or neglect by a caregiver, before the age of 17 years.[2] Exposure to developmental trauma and its effects on the child-caregiver relationship have been shown to negatively impact children's emotional, relational, cognitive, behavioral, and neurobiological development.[3] Considering the wide-ranging effects and the absence of a psychiatric diagnosis for developmental trauma, the symptoms and behaviors expressed by children with histories of abuse and neglect are often misdiagnosed or undiagnosed, and are therefore not always provided with the appropriate interventions to support their needs.[4,5] DTD has been proposed as an additional psychiatric diagnosis to the existing PTSD diagnosis in order to better assess and address the symptomology of developmental trauma.[5,6] This chapter aims to provide a broad-strokes introduction to students and practitioners that are new to the field of trauma studies and interventions, and to serve as a starting point for further learning and professional development.

Conceptualizing Trauma

The term *trauma* typically refers to an individual's response to a perceived or actual life-threatening event that overwhelms a person's usual mechanisms of adaptation and results in ongoing physiological, psychological, and relational effects that continue to manifest after the event is over.[7] Traumatic events (or experiences) can be organized into 2 main categories: single incident trauma and complex trauma.[8] *Single incident trauma* refers to events that are unexpected and out of the norm, such as injury, threat of injury, or death resulting from experiences of or exposure to natural disasters, car accidents, terrorist attacks, or violent crime.[8] *Complex trauma* typically occurs within the context of multiple or ongoing interpersonal victimizations (ie, harm inflicted by one person onto another), such as: direct or indirect exposure to interpersonal or domestic violence; physical, sexual, and emotional abuse; medical or emotional neglect; or the compounding effects of structural violence and injustices resulting from racism, cisheterosexism, settler colonialism, and other harmful systems of oppression.[8,9]

Developmental trauma is often conceptualized within the context of complex trauma, specifically referring to interpersonal victimization within the context of caregiver-child relationships, such as: physical, sexual, or emotional abuse; emotional, physical, or medical neglect/maltreatment; witnessing interpersonal violence; caregiver impairment; and traumatic separation from caregivers.[8,10] The use of the term "developmental" reflects both the timing of an individual's experiences of complex traumatic experiences in the early developmental stages of their lives and the impact of those experiences on the individual's social, emotional, cognitive, and neurobiological development through adolescence and adulthood.[10,11] Developmental trauma can occur as a result of direct victimization by a caregiver or by witnessing the victimization of a sibling, other child, or other caregiver. This form of victimization can disrupt the formation and maintenance of secure attachment between caregiver and child, which can in turn impact the child's internal sense of safety, self-regulation skills, identity development, and quality of relationships.[5]

DIAGNOSING TRAUMA DISORDERS IN CHILDREN AND ADOLESCENTS

Despite the high rate of children who have been exposed to interpersonal victimization and our increased understanding of the effects of developmental trauma on children's functioning and developmental trajectories, a formal psychiatric diagnosis for developmental trauma does not yet exist as of the publishing of this book.[5] PTSD remains the only psychiatric diagnosis for trauma-related symptoms and focuses on trauma symptom manifestation following exposure to a single incident trauma.[6,12] DTD has been proposed as an additional psychiatric diagnosis that could better capture the symptomology of children and adolescents who have experienced developmental trauma, and thus also provide improved intervention outcomes as a result of more comprehensive and appropriate assessment.[5,6,13]

In order to meet the diagnostic criteria for PTSD, an individual must have experienced or witnessed a single incident traumatic event and demostrate symptoms across 4 symptom clusters.[12] The symptom categories include: intrusion symptoms (ie, intrusive memories and dreams related to the traumatic event), avoidance symptoms (ie, avoiding internal reminders such as memories and thoughts or external reminders such as people or places related to the traumatic event), altered cognitions and mood (ie, persistant negative thoughts about self or negative emotional state), and hypervigilance (ie, increased anxiety, exaggerated startle response, and irritability).[8] The diagnostic criteria are modified for children ages 6 years and under, recognizing some of the ways in which trauma symptoms may present differently in children. For example, intrusive symptoms may manifest through the re-enactment of traumatic experiences during play or recurring nightmares with content that may not directly relate to traumatic experiences; avoidance symptoms may look like social withdrawal; and hypervigilance may look like extreme temper tantrums.[14]

Due to diversity in the presentation of trauma symptoms, overlap with other conditions, and the absence of a developmentally-specific trauma disorder (such as the proposed DTD), children affected by developmental trauma are often undiagnosed, misdiagnosed, or dually diagnosed with other psychiatric disorders such as anxiety, depression, attention deficit hyperactivity disorder, or oppositional defiant disorder.[15] Developmental trauma can impact children's affect presentation and behavior, concentration and executive functioning, self-concept and efficacy, cognitive patterns, and social and relational skills. At home, this may manifest as a child having frequent and seemingly unprompted meltdowns, spending most of their time alone in their room, engaging in self-harming behaviors, engaging in hypersexualized or aggressive forms of play, or not being able to complete their familial and household duties. At school, it could be a child having difficulty sitting still, excessive fatigue, difficulty concentrating on school work, anger outbursts, difficulty making and keeping friends, withdrawn behavior, or lower academic performance.[16]

When assessed without the lens of developmental trauma, these symptoms may meet the criteria for other psychiatric diagnoses; therefore, treatment may be focused on modifying those behaviors rather than addressing the underlying sypmtoms of trauma and disrupted attachment. Without standardized diagnostic criteria for developmental trauma, many children are left without the necessary trauma-focused support they need for both intrapersonal and interpersonal healing.[14] In many cases, unfortunately, children are labeled by parents, teachers, and even medical and mental health professionals as defiant, oppositional, delinquent, or problematic, and are consequently treated with punitive or isolationary approaches. The proposed DTD offers a supplemental framework to the existing PTSD diagnostic criteria that encompasses the nuanced and often misdiagnosed manifestation of developmental trauma symptoms amongst children and adolescents.[4,5]

In contrast to the focus on single incident trauma in the assessment and diagnosis of PTSD, the first criterion of the proposed DTD includes severe or repeating exposure to interpersonal victimization and traumatic disruption of protective caregiving.[13] Symptoms are then organized into 3 domains: emotion and somatic dysregulation (including impaired access or expression of emotions or somatic feelings), attentional or behavioral dysregulation (including preoccupation with threat and maladaptive self-soothing), and self and interpersonal dysregulation (including self-loathing, attachment insecurity, and reactive aggression).[13] While there are similarities between the diagnostic criteria for PTSD and DTD, DTD expands the focus on trauma-related dysregulation across children's psychological, somatic, cognitive, and relational functioning.[4]

INTERVENTIONS FOR DEVELOPMENTAL TRAUMA

The accurate assessment and diagnosis of trauma-related symptoms is central to developing and implementing appropriate clinical interventions.[13] The unique constellation and presentation of PTSD or DTD symptoms can inform which treatment approaches may be most beneficial to children and their family systems at different stages of treatment. The interpersonal nature of developmental trauma and its occurance in early years of development highlight the importance of selecting interventions that engage the child and caregiver when appropriate, while also providing developmentally appropriate opportunities for expression and connection. Interventions such as Parent-Child Psychotherapy and Parent-Child Interaction Therapy focus on improving caregiver-child relationships through increased caregiver attunement, emotion regulation, communication, and social skills.[17,18] The Attachment, Regulation, and Competency (ARC) framework facilitates personal relational healing within the family system and focuses on developing attunement and co-regulation skills by engaging children and their caregivers in cognitive, relational, and behavioral interventions.[19]

Play-based and expressive interventions, such as Sensory Motor Arousal Regulation Treatment (SMART), support children, adolescents, and caregivers by strengthening emotion and interpersonal regulation skills through sensory focused play.[20] Child-Centered Play Therapy and expressive art interventions can provide children and adolescents with opportunities for developmentally appropriate exploration, processing, and communication.[21] These forms of therapy create space for nonverbal expression, thereby allowing children and adolescents to engage in healing through the intuitive language of play and art. Trauma-informed, body-oriented interventions for children and adolescents, such as yoga, mindfulness, and dance, can increase self-awareness and regulation skills and improve emotional and behavioral functioning.[22,23] Animal-assisted therapies, such as equine-assisted psychotherapy, can nurture feelings of trust and self-worth and increase self-regulation and co-regulation skills through children and adolescents' relationships with their animal partner.[19,24]

Cognitive and behavioral therapeutic modalities have also been used as trauma interventions for adolescents and adults, including Cognitive Behavioral Therapy, Cognitive Processing Therapy, and Prolonged Exposure Therapy.[25] Trauma-Focused Cognitive Behavioral Therapy (TF-CBT) and Cognitive Behavioral Intervention for Trauma in Schools (CBITS) are among the most extensively researched cognitive-behavioral interventions for children and adolescents who have experienced trauma.[15] Both TF-CBT and CBITS are structured, short-term interventions (between 8 and 25 sessions) that incorporate self-regulation skills, cognitive behavioral techniques, psychoeducation, and collaboration with adults (eg, caregivers or educators) to reduce trauma symptoms.[25,26]

KEY POINTS

1. Developmental trauma refers to interpersonal victimization within the context of caregiver-child relationships, including maltreatment, abuse, and neglect.

2. Developmental trauma can impact children's affect presentation, behavior, executive functioning, self-concept, cognitive patterns, interpersonal skills, and neurobiological development.

3. Developmental trauma symptom domains include: emotion and somatic dysregulation, attentional or behavioral dysregulation, and self and interpersonal dysregulation.

4. Appropriate interventions engage the child and caregiver when appropriate and provide opportunities for expression, regulation, and connection.

REFERENCES

1. Bethell CD, Davis MB, Gombojav N, Stumbo S, Powers K. A national and across state profile on adverse childhood experiences among children and possibilities to heal and thrive. Johns Hopkins Bloomberg School of Public Health. 2017. https://www.cahmi.org/docs/default-source/resources/issue-brief-a-nation-al-and-across-state-profile-on-adverse-childhood-experiences-among-children-and-possibilities-to-heal-and-thrive-(2017).pdf?sfvrsn=18ba657f_0

2. Fortson BL, Klevens J, Merrick MT, Gilbert LK, Alexander SP. Preventing child abuse and neglect: a technical package for policy, norm, and programmatic activities. National Center for Injury Prevention and Control; Centers for Disease Control and Prevention. 2016. https://www.cdc.gov/violenceprevention/pdf/can-prevention-technical-package.pdf

3. Spinazzola J, van der Kolk B, Ford JD. When nowhere is safe: interpersonal trauma and attachment adversity as antecedents of posttraumatic stress disorder and developmental trauma disorder. *J Trauma Stress.* 2018;31(5):631-642. doi:10.1002/jts.22320

4. Ford JD, Spinazzola J, van der Kolk BA, Chan G. Toward an empirically based Developmental Trauma Disorder diagnosis and semi-structured interview for children: the DTD field trial replication. *Acta Psychiatr Scand.* 2022; 145(6):628–39. doi:10.1111/acps.13424

5. Ford JD, Spinazzola J, van der Kolk B, et al. Toward an empirically based developmental trauma disorder diagnosis for children: factor structure, item characteristics, reliability, and validity of the Developmental Trauma Disorder Semi-Structured Interview. *J Clin Psychiatry.* 2018;79(5):17m11675. doi:10.4088/JCP.17m11675

6. van der Kolk BA, Pynoos RS, Cicchetti D, et al. Proposal to include a developmental trauma disorder diagnosis for children and adolescents in DSM-V. 2009; Unpublished manuscript. http://www.cathymalchiodi. com/dtd_nctsn. pdf

7. Herman J. *Trauma and Recovery*. Basic Books; 1997.

8. Ford JD, Courtois CA. Defining and understanding complex trauma and complex traumatic stress disorders. In: *Treating Complex Traumatic Stress Disorders*. The Guilford Press; 2014.

9. Saleem FT, Anderson RE, Monnica W. Addressing the "myth" of racial trauma: developmental and ecological considerations for youth of color. *Clin Child Fam Psychol Rev.* 2020;23(1):1-14. doi:10.1007/s10567-019-00304-1

10. Spinazzola J, van der Kolk B, Ford JD. Developmental trauma disorder: a legacy of attachment trauma in victimized children. *J Trauma Stress.* 2021;34(4):711-720. doi:10.1002/jts.22697

11. Perry BD. Examining child maltreatment through a neurodevelopmental lens: clinical applications of the neurosequential model of therapeutics. *J Loss Trauma.* 2009;14(4):240-255. doi:10.1080/15325020903004350

12. American Psychiatric Association. *Diagnostic and Statistical Manual of Mental Disorders.* 5th ed. American Psychiatric Publishing; 2022.

13. Ford JD. Why we need a developmentally appropriate trauma diagnosis for children: a 10-year update on developmental trauma disorder. *J Child Adolesc Trauma.* 2021;16(2):403-418. doi:10.1007/s40653-021-00415-4

14. D'Andrea W, Ford J, Stolbach B, Spinazzola J, van der Kolk BA. Understanding interpersonal trauma in children: why we need a developmentally appropriate trauma diagnosis. *Am Orthopsychiatry.* 2012;82(2):187-200. doi:10.1111/j.1939-0025.2012.01154.x

15. Chafouleas SM, Koriakin TA, Roundfield KD, Overstreet S. Addressing childhood trauma in school settings: a framework for evidence-based practice. *School Ment Health.* 2019;11(1):40-53. doi:10.1007/s12310-018-9256-5

16. Ford JD, Cloitre M. Best practices in psychotherapy for children and adolescents. In: Courtois CA, Ford JD, eds. *Treating Complex Traumatic Stress Disorders*. The Guilford Press; 2014.

17. Hagan MJ, Browne DT, Sulik M, Ippen CG, Bush N, Lieberman AF. Parent and child trauma symptoms during child-parent psychotherapy: a prospective cohort study of dyadic change. *J Trauma Stress.* 2017;30(6):690-697. doi:10.1002/jts.22240

18. Thomas R, Zimmer-Gembeck MJ. Parent–child interaction therapy: an evidence-based treatment for child maltreatment. *Child Maltreatment.* 2012;17(3):253–266. doi:10.1177/1077559512459555

19. Blaustein ME, Kinniburgh KM. Attachment, self-regulation, and competency (ARC). In: Landolt MA, Cloitre M, Schnyder U, eds. *Evidence-Based Treatments for Trauma Related Disorders in Children and Adolescents.* Springer International Publishing; 2017.

20. Warner E, Spinazzola J, Wescott A, Gunn C, Hodgdon H. The body can change the score: empirical support for somatic regulation in the treatment of traumatized adolescents. *J Child Adolesc Trauma.* 2014;7(4):237–246. doi:10.1007/s40653-014-0030-z

21. Ray DC, Burgin E, Gutierrez D, Ceballos P, Lindo N. Child-centered play therapy and adverse childhood experiences: a randomized controlled trial. *J Couns Dev.* 2022;100(2):134-145. doi:10.1002/jcad.12412

22. Razza RA, Uveges Linsner R, Bergen-Cico D, Carlson E, Reid S. The feasibility and effectiveness of mindful yoga for preschoolers exposed to high levels of trauma. *J Child Fam Stud.* 2020;29(1):82-93. doi:10.1007/s10826-019-01582-7

23. Beltran M, Brown-Elhillali AN, Held AR, et al. Yoga-based psychotherapy groups for boys exposed to trauma in urban settings. *Altern Ther Health Med.* 2016;22(1):39-46.

24. Naste TM, Price M, Karol J, et al. Equine facilitated therapy for complex trauma (EFT-CT). *J Child Adolesc Trauma.* 2018;11(3):289-303. doi:10.1007/s40653-017-0187-3

25. Rudd BN, Last BS, Gregor C, et al. Benchmarking treatment effectiveness of community delivered trauma focused cognitive behavioral therapy. *Am J Community Psychol.* 2019;64(3-4):438-450. doi:10.1002/ajcp.12370

26. Allison AC, Ferreira RJ. Implementing cognitive behavioral intervention for trauma in schools (cbits) with latino youth. *Child Adolesc Soc Work J.* 2017; 34(2):181-189. doi:10.1007/s10560-016-0486-9

Chapter 2

Neuropsychological Implications of Child Maltreatment

Andrew Davis, PhD

Tania E. Morales Zelaya, MA, Ball State University

Stevie B. Knight, MA, Ball State University

Megan E. Slagel, MA, Ball State University

Brian Cheline, MA, Ball State University

Objectives

After reading this chapter, the reader will be able to:

1. *Identify the potential immediate and long-term neurological changes that are associated with child maltreatment.*

2. *Describe the role of the neuroendocrine system, specifically the Hypothalamic-Pituitary-Adrenal (HPA) axis in child maltreatment and how it places children at risk for poor outcomes.*

3. *Understand the need to refer maltreated children, and some adults, for neuropsychological testing when they are experiencing cognitive difficulties.*

Background and Significance

Child abuse and neglect, henceforth referred to as child maltreatment, has a pervasive and devastating effect on the child, their family, and the community. Child maltreatment can potentially have immediate and long-lasting effects on a child's developing central nervous system. A 2018 meta-analysis indicated a relationship between brain structures and maltreatment-related post-traumatic stress disorder (PTSD).[1] These authors concluded that the most noteworthy structural differences were seen in reduced brain volumes in the amygdala, cerebellum, corpus callosum, hippocampus, and total cerebral volume. These areas of the brain are associated with a host of cognitive and academic functions including emotions, memory, motor functioning, executive functioning, and reading. The widespread neurological morphological concerns demonstrate the array of difficulties with which children who experience child maltreatment can present, with possible long-term implications.

Neurodevelopmental aberrations have a synergistic relationship with the child's environment (eg, school, home, community) which can result in repercussions for multiple systems in the child's life. As such, neurodevelopmental concerns represent a longitudinal risk factor for difficulty with academic, social, emotional, psychiatric, and vocational functioning, though not all children who experience maltreatment have these outcomes. A neuropsychological perspective represents an ideal lens through which to view these potential negative outcomes associated with child maltreatment. Neuropsychology refers to the integration of neurological (ie, central nervous system functioning) and psychological (eg, social, emotional, and behavioral functioning) factors that typically are assessed through performance-based tests, observation, and objective rating scales in a variety of functional domains. These domains include memory, attention, executive functioning, visual-spatial abilities, sensory-motor, language, academic abilities, adaptive functions (ie, activities of daily living), and social-emotional functions. When combined with a review of the patient's history (eg, medical, educational, legal, vocational, psychosocial), the clinical neuropsychologist is able to use hypothesis testing to make differential diagnostic determinations, determine functional capacity, and provide recommendations for treatment, accommodations, and interventions across multiple settings.

NEUROLOGICAL MORPHOLOGICAL CHANGES ASSOCIATED WITH CHILD MALTREATMENT

In addition to the morphological changes associated with external physical forces (eg, traumatic brain injuries), intracranial insults (eg, a cerebral vascular accident), and in the presence of neurodegenerative conditions (eg, metachromatic leukodystrophy or multiple sclerosis), emerging research shows that emotional trauma can also result in morphological changes.[1] Despite well-known neural plasticity mechanisms that occur in childhood compared to adulthood, morphological changes to the brain during childhood can interrupt neurodevelopmental stages and interfere with or delay the acquisition of milestones, potentially leading to lifelong consequences. Evolutionary theorists suggest that structural changes occur via a compensating mechanism to enable survival despite living in threatening conditions,[2,3] a phenomenon that has been referred to as "phenotypic plasticity." This term highlights the adaptive response of individuals to stressful, non-optimal environments that influence development.[3]

Perhaps the most well-studied structures associated with child maltreatment include the limbic system (eg, the hippocampus and amygdala) and the anterior cingulate cortex (ACC). The limbic system, like many brain areas, is multifunctional and involved with memory and emotion. Meta-analytic results documented a reduced bilateral hippocampal volume among adults with childhood maltreatment-related PTSD relative to healthy controls.[4] In children, however, the amygdala and hippocampus volumes were comparable to their healthy control counterparts, which is likely an indication of the effects of child maltreatment on neurodevelopment that become visible in adulthood.[4] This type of study shows that potential neurological changes associated with child maltreatment may not emerge until later in life and highlights the need for medical professionals to inquire of adult patients about a history of child maltreatment. Additional studies have reported reduced cortical thickness (ie, a measure of the amount of neural tissue) in the right ventral ACC, superior frontal gyrus, and anterior orbitofrontal cortex (OFC) in children with a history of maltreatment.[5] A 2021 study[6] also reported negative associations between child maltreatment and volume of the right amygdala, anterior hippocampus, and bilateral cornu ammonis subfield among participants with a history of child maltreatment and major depressive disorder (MDD). More importantly, only the history of child maltreatment was related to their volumetric findings; neither the diagnosis of MDD nor history of treatment with antidepressants showed significant effects.[6] Child maltreatment is also associated with reduced cerebellar volumes bilaterally.[7] Cerebellar volume was positively associated with age of onset of child maltreatment and negatively correlated with the duration of trauma associated with PTSD.[7]

Maltreatment has also been associated with reduced white matter integrity in the left arcuate fasciculus, and reduced gray matter density among areas responsible for visual perception, discrimination, and integration, the left and right lingual gyrus, and the left occipital pole, secondary visual cortex, and the left inferior longitudinal fasciculus.[5,8,9] Functional magnetic resonance imaging (fMRI) data also suggests patterns of brain utilization among adults with a history of childhood maltreatment.

While completing a psychosocial stress task, participants with a history of child maltreatment demonstrated increased activation in the dorsolateral prefrontal cortex (dlPFC), insula, and precuneus, along with decreased activation in the ventromedial prefrontal cortex (vmPFC).[10]

The increased consideration of biomarkers in the literature suggests that this represents an important aspect of practice in the diagnosis of psychiatric conditions. As neuroimaging research continues to progress and be used in clinical practice, the identification of morphological findings may someday help providers with early identification of behavioral concerns associated with child maltreatment. At this point, however, there is too much overlap in functional neuroanatomical changes or disturbance between multiple conditions, which leads neuroimaging to be better suited for some conditions than others. For a variety of reasons, children and parents or caregivers are often reluctant to report maltreatment to health care providers; therefore, looking for biomarkers or clinical indicators of maltreatment may help providers in identifying the presence of such.

Child maltreatment has long been considered a risk factor for the presence of a myriad of psychiatric disorders in adulthood, including depression,[6,11,12] anxiety,[12] PTSD,[13-15] borderline personality disorder,[16] and bipolar disorder.[17,18] Data overwhelmingly suggests that beyond being a risk factor, the structural and functional changes associated with child maltreatment underlie psychiatric illness via epigenetic factors. The research suggests the presence of disrupted connectivity in the resting-state networks in individuals with depression and a history of child maltreatment.[19] He et al[11] found decreasing levels of peripheral blood miR-9 among those with more severe childhood maltreatment and depressive symptoms which overlapped with patterns of connectivity in the prefrontal-parietal-striatum and limbic system. The data clearly suggests a strong role of miRNA in the expression of psychopathology, including schizophrenia, depression, bipolar disorder, PTSD, and anxiety. These types of findings also highlight the relationship of child maltreatment to epigenetics (ie, the way environment can impact a person's genetics).

The neurological effects of child maltreatment appear to diffuse and impact several functional brain areas associated with cognitive, social, emotional, behavioral, and academic functioning and also appear to represent a lifelong risk factor for the development of these concerns. A longitudinal study[20] found childhood maltreatment to be associated with increases in resting-state functional connectivity (rsFC) in widespread networks, including the default mode, dorsal attention, and frontoparietal networks. From the initial data collection point to the second collection point (approximately 2.5 years after), there was a shift in increased rsFC from subcortical and sensory circuitry to primarily frontal circuitry at T2. The study concluded that childhood maltreatment is associated with a different neurodevelopmental trajectory that likely underlies the presence of depression and substance use disorders among adolescents.[20] As these networks can be associated with the development of psychopathology, they showcase the brain mechanisms that can increase the risk of developing psychopathology in individuals with a history of childhood maltreatment.

NEUROENDOCRINE EFFECTS OF CHILD MALTREATMENT

A wealth of evidence indicates that early experiences of child maltreatment may have long-lasting consequences on physiological and psychological outcomes in adulthood. Adverse childhood experiences, including maltreatment, are among the primary contributors to poor mental health outcomes later in life.[21,22] Research suggests that different forms of maltreatment, occurring at any stage of development, put children at greater risk for developing psychiatric illnesses characterized by more serious symptomology and comorbidity as well as a more severe disease course marked by higher medication dosages, increased suicidal behavior, and more frequent hospitalizations.[23,24]

The underlying etiology of such mental health concerns is multifactorial; however, research related to the role of the neuroendocrine system, particularly the HPA axis, suggests it plays a critical role in the underlying pathophysiology.

The neuroendocrine system is a communication mechanism that involves multiple glands in the brain and throughout the rest of the body. Primarily, it maintains homeostasis through a network of pathways used to communicate with various systems of the body via chemical messengers called hormones.[25] Child maltreatment, through the initiation of a stress response, can have an immediate and chronic maladaptive effect on the neuroendocrine system. In the presence of a perceived stressor, the human body initiates a stress response that regulates and adapts physiological processes toward the maintenance of homeostasis.[25] The HPA axis plays a major role in this homeostatic response through the initiation of a cascade of endocrine reactions that allow for physiological adaptation by modulating processes including metabolism, reproductive processes, immune responses, and the autonomic nervous system.[25] Understanding how the HPA axis contributes to the stress response in the absence of chronic stress or maltreatment informs recognition of its role in maltreatment and the development of maladaptive sequelae.

Dysregulation of the HPA axis is associated with the development of a number of physiological and psychiatric concerns. The HPA axis regulates through a negative feedback loop that is responsive to the dose and duration of exposure to plasma-level glucocorticoids (GC), such as cortisol.[26] When circulatory cortisol levels are too high, signals are sent to the hypothalamus and the hippocampus to inhibit further HPA axis activation.[25,27] However, in the presence of chronic stress or maltreatment, this feedback loop may be impaired due to prolonged hyperactivity of the amygdala and reduced activity of the hippocampus (part of the limbic system, suggesting involvement of memory and emotion).[28,29] There is a lack of consensus regarding the impact of such impairment, as some research suggests that exposure to child maltreatment results in overactivity of the HPA axis and excessive serum levels of cortisol (ie, hypercortisolism), while others demonstrate a blunted cortisol response during peak and recovery phases of acute stress with accompanying overall hypocortisolism.[30,31] Increasing research suggests that both hypercortisolism and hypocortisolism may be a result depending on the type, severity, and frequency of maltreatment experienced. Marques-Feixa et al[32] found that child maltreatment and serum cortisol levels have a dose-response relationship such that those who experience more severe maltreatment or more frequent exposure to it demonstrate higher overall diurnal cortisol levels and a diminished release of cortisol in response to an acute stressor. They also found that higher doses of maltreatment were associated with greater perceived anxiety.[32] Turner et al[33] suggested patterns of hyperactivity and hypoactivity are associated with different psychiatric outcomes.

As a result of the neuroendocrine effects of childhood maltreatment, individuals may suffer from neurophysiological effects in adulthood. Basu et al[34] analyzed 40 publications related to childhood maltreatment, cardiovascular disease, and type 2 diabetes and found that most studies identified a significant relationship among these variables. The majority of studies suggested that the more instances of maltreatment a child experiences, the more likely individuals are to have cardiometabolic diseases. Specifically, 91.7% of the studies that examined childhood maltreatment and cardiovascular disease found a significant relationship. 61.5% found a relationship between increased blood pressure or hypertension and childhood maltreatment, and 88.2% found a relationship with diabetes.[34] Given the potential neurological implications of these conditions (eg, cerebrovascular disease), it is important for practitioners to consider that negative health consequences that are not typically considered "neurological" in nature still have the potential to interfere with cognition, academics, and other functional activities.

COGNITIVE EFFECTS OF CHILDHOOD MALTREATMENT

Given the literature regarding morphological and neuroendocrine changes associated with child maltreatment, corresponding neurocognitive deficits can be presumed present in children who have experienced maltreatment. There is, however, not a simple 1:1 correlation between acquired brain changes and behavioral changes, as the psychosocial variables associated with child maltreatment can also produce cognitive deficits that have a psychogenic etiology. For example, children who experience depression[35-38] or anxiety[35-37] are likely to present with attention, concentration, and memory deficits. Children who experience maltreatment are also statistically more likely to come from low-income homes,[39,40] and low socioeconomic status (SES) is correlated to lower scores on general tests of intellectual functioning[41,42] as well as for psychopathology.[43] This highlights the need to interpret IQ tests with caution, as clinicians need to carefully consider the impact of SES and other demographic factors; in essence, children from lower SES backgrounds may have had less exposure to the material and types of problems present on IQ tests. Additionally, it is essential to consider psychopathology as manifesting when differences are present from the person's culture (not deviant from the majority culture), rendering a thorough assessment of the child's culture and level of acculturation a key component of a neuropsychological evaluation. In sum, children who experience maltreatment are likely to have a number of individual risk (and possible resilience) factors which can produce a heterogeneous cognitive profile when this population is studied as a group. An additional complicating factor in predicting the cognitive sequelae of childhood maltreatment is the plethora of literature demonstrating that childhood maltreatment impacts developmental, neurocognitive, and psychiatric conditions at the time of abuse and into adulthood.[44-49] Given these factors, children with a history of maltreatment are likely to benefit from individual assessments to determine the best accommodations and interventions. Neuropsychological assessments are likely to be the most comprehensive, but at a minimum, these factors should be considered in children who are referred for special education evaluation (eg, psychoeducational testing). It is also possible that cognitive,[50] social-emotional,[51,52] behavioral,[53] and academic problems[54] may not manifest until years after the trauma. Common areas of neurocognitive functioning assessed during a neuropsychological evaluation include intelligence, executive functioning, memory, attention, language, visuospatial abilities, and motor functioning.

INTELLIGENCE

Intelligence is a multifaceted construct with an array of definitions. Intelligence tests typically measure a variety of different constructs and provide composite scores (eg, IQ scores) that represent a general estimate of the patient's ability to solve problems compared to their same-aged peers. Intelligence tests (and virtually all neuropsychological measures) are significantly influenced by a number of noninherent factors including culture, SES, parental level of education, and stereotype threat, again highlighting the caution providers should take in interpreting IQ scores as a measure of a child's "innate" ability or potential.[55-57]

In Kavanaugh et al's[48] review of literature regarding the neurocognitive profiles in individuals who experienced childhood maltreatment, they consistently found that children who have experienced maltreatment have lower intellectual functioning compared to the control group. Despite lower intellectual functioning compared to the control group, results suggest that IQ still largely falls within the average to below average range. It is important to consider that most measures of intellectual functioning do not measure all neurocognitive functions (eg, executive functions, memory). In some cases, while intelligence tests measure linguistic and visual problem solving, they do not fully explore the basic aspects of these functions (eg, naming, verbal fluency). As such, the findings that many children with a history of maltreatment do not have significantly lower IQ scores does not mean they do not have other areas of cognitive concern, which is one of the reasons a comprehensive neuropsychological assessment can be helpful.

EXECUTIVE FUNCTIONING

Executive functioning has been defined in a variety of ways, including functions that contribute to independent, purposeful, and self-directed behaviors[58] that enable the individual to modulate, control, and organize their behavior for the purpose of making decisions and problem solving in novel situations.[59] Research has found impairments in executive functioning for children who have experienced maltreatment compared to healthy controls; however, the impairments do not demonstrate a unique profile and instead suggest general weaknesses across several domains. Irigaray et al[46] examined 17 research articles investigating the association between cognitive functioning and childhood maltreatment and found that 63.6% of the articles noted deficits in problem solving, planning, mental flexibility, inhibition, information processing, and abstract reasoning that extended into adulthood. Similar findings occurred in other studies, demonstrating deficits in inhibitory control,[44,45,50] planning and organizing,[47,60] and cognitive flexibility.[60,61] This can be related to the early findings discussing prefrontal cortex concerns (ie, the area of the brain where executive functioning is primarily "housed").

MEMORY

Given the diffuse neural network that is engaged during memory-based functions, it is unsurprising that memory is adversely impacted by childhood maltreatment. Navalta et al[62] conducted a linear regression analysis of college-aged women that indicated that for each year of abuse, there was a 2.4% reduction in short-term memory, a 2% reduction in verbal memory, a 1.9% reduction in visual memory, and an overall 2.3% reduction in global memory. De Bellis et al[45] found that children who suffered from maltreatment (with or without a PTSD diagnosis) performed significantly worse on measures of memory, and sexual abuse was associated with greater deficits. Similarly, Kavanaugh et al[48] found that children and adolescents who experienced maltreatment demonstrate verbal and visual memory weaknesses, with the presence of sexual abuse being more strongly correlated. Irigaray et al[46] also found that in 66.7% of the articles they examined, children and adults with a history of childhood maltreatment showed impairment in various types of memory, such as working memory and verbal episodic memory.

LANGUAGE

Research has demonstrated inconsistent findings on language abilities following childhood maltreatment. A longitudinal study[63] found that children with a history of abuse, despite starting with similar receptive language skills, developed at a significantly slower rate and peaked in their skills at an earlier age than their non-abused peers. Similarly, multiple studies[45,46,60,64] have found that abuse and maltreatment have significant negative impacts on receptive and expressive language. The impact of childhood maltreatment on language is extremely important given the impact that language has on a variety of functions, including academics.[65] Poor academics can increase the child's likelihood of dropping out of school, engaging in criminal activity, becoming incarcerated, or becoming homeless[54,66]; therefore, it is imperative that language be assessed if childhood maltreatment is present.

CONCLUSION

Childhood maltreatment negatively impacts the neurodevelopmental process in children and represents a salient risk factor for the development of adult pathology. Morphological brain changes following child maltreatment are evident in the literature, as are neuroendocrine concerns. Deficits can occur in various functional domains that are important for acquisition of academic, social, and emotional abilities, including neurocognitive concerns in intellectual functioning, executive functioning, memory, and language. While deficits in these areas are consistently shown in the literature, similar to neuroimaging findings, a specific neuropsychological profile is not salient. Neurocognitive deficits may be associated with the type, severity, duration, and frequency of maltreatment as well as the period of development during which maltreatment occurred and the presence of comorbid conditions. The relationship between childhood maltreatment and psychological sequelae is indicative of lifelong problems that may vary in presentation and severity across individuals. Despite the vast difference between forms of abuse and neglect, there seems to be substantial overlap between mental health disorders that commonly occur following maltreatment. Providers should be aware of the potential neurological and psychological outcomes associated with child maltreatment to facilitate identification and treatment.

KEY POINTS

1. Child maltreatment has the potential to substantially interfere with neurodevelopment in several different domains.

2. The effects of child maltreatment may not manifest until later in life, which suggests that even in the absence of obvious features, providers should continue to ask all patients about child maltreatment.

3. When child maltreatment is found, in addition to following state and federal reporting guidelines, providers are encouraged to consider assessment for the domains discussed in this chapter as they can all interfere with functioning.

REFERENCES

1. Killion B, Weyandt L. Brain structure in childhood maltreatment-related PTSD across the lifespan: a systemic review. *Appl Neuropsychol Child.* 2020;9(1):68-82. doi:10.1080/21622965.2018.1515076 PMID:30351191

2. Gibb BE, Schofield CA, Coles ME. Reported history of childhood abuse and young adults' information-processing biases for facial displays of emotion. *Child Maltreat.* 2009;14(2):148-156. doi:10.1177/1077559508326358

3. Belsky J, Pluess M. Beyond risk, resilience, and dysregulation: phenotypic plasticity and human development. *Dev Psychopathol.* 2013;25(4 Pt 2):1243-1261. doi:10.1017/S095457941300059X

4. Woon FL, Hedges DW. Hippocampal and amygdala volumes in children and adults with childhood maltreatment-related posttraumatic stress disorder: a meta-analysis. *Hippocampus.* 2008;18(8):729-736. doi:10.1002/hipo.20437

5. Kelly PA, Viding E, Wallace GL, et al. Cortical thickness, surface area, and gyrification abnormalities in children exposed to maltreatment: neural markers of vulnerability? *Biol Psychiatry.* 2013;74(11):845-852. doi:10.1016/j.biopsych.2013.06.020

6. Aghamohammadi-Sereshki A, Coupland NJ, Silverstone PH, et al. Effects of childhood adversity on the volumes of the amygdala subnuclei and hippocampal subfields in individuals with major depressive disorder. *J Psychiatry Neurosci.* 2021;46(1):E186-E195. doi:10.1503/jpn.200034

7. De Bellis MD, Kuchibhatla M. Cerebellar volumes in pediatric maltreatment-related posttraumatic stress disorder. *Biol Psychiatry.* 2006;60(7):697-703. doi:10.1016/j.biopsych.2006.04.035

8. Choi J, Jeong B, Rohan ML, Polcari AM, Teicher MH. Preliminary evidence for white matter tract abnormalities in young adults exposed to parental verbal abuse. *Biol Psychiatry.* 2009;65(3):227-234. doi:10.1016/j.biopsych.2008.06.022

9. Tomoda A, Polcari A, Anderson CM, Teicher MH. Reduced visual cortex gray matter volume and thickness in young adults who witnessed domestic violence during childhood. *PLoS One*. 2012;7(12):e52528. doi:10.1371/journal.pone.0052528

10. Zhong X, Ming Q, Dong D, et al. Childhood maltreatment experience influences neural response to psychosocial stress in adults: an fMRI study. *Front Psychol*. 2019;10:2961. doi:10.3389/fpsyg.2019.02961

11. He C, Bai Y, Wang Z, et al. Identification of microRNA-9 linking the effects of childhood maltreatment on depression using amygdala connectivity. *NeuroImage*. 2021;224:117428. doi:10.1016/j.neuroimage.2020.117428 PMID:33038536

12. Heim C, Nemeroff CB. The role of childhood trauma in the neurobiology of mood and anxiety disorders: preclinical and clinical studies. *Biol Psychiatry*. 2001;49(12):1023-1039. doi:10.1016/s0006-3223(01)01157-x

13. Hovens JG, Giltay EJ, Spinhoven P, van Hemert AM, Penninx BW. Impact of childhood life events and childhood trauma on the onset and recurrence of depressive and anxiety disorders. *J Clin Psychiatry*. 2015;76(7):931-938. doi:10.4088/JCP.14m09135

14. Breslau N, Koenen KC, Luo Z, et al. Childhood maltreatment, juvenile disorders and adult post-traumatic stress disorder: a prospective investigation. *Psychol Med*. 2014;44(9):1937-1945. doi:10.1017/S0033291713002651

15. Wieck A, Grassi-Oliveira R, Hartmann do Prado C, Teixeira AL, Bauer ME. Neuroimmunoendocrine interactions in post-traumatic stress disorder: focus on long-term implications of childhood maltreatment. *Neuroimmunomodulation*. 2014;21:145-151. doi:10.1159/000356552

16. Cattane N, Rossi R, Lanfredi M, Cattaneo A. Borderline personality disorder and childhood trauma: exploring the affected biological systems and mechanisms. *BMC Psychiatry*. 2017;17(1):221. doi:10.1186/s12888-017-1383-2

17. Watson S, Gallagher P, Dougall D, et al. Childhood trauma in bipolar disorder. *Aust N Z J Psychiatry*. 2014;48(6):564-570. doi:10.1177/0004867413516681

18. Garno JL, Goldberg JF, Ramirez PM, Ritzler BA. Impact of childhood abuse on the clinical course of bipolar disorder. *Br J Psychiatry*. 2005;186(2):121-125. doi:10.1192/bjp.186.2.121

19. Yu M, Linn KA, Shinohara RT, et al. Childhood trauma history is linked to abnormal brain connectivity in major depression. *Proc Natl Acad Sci USA*. 2019;116:8582-8590. doi:10.1073/pnas.1900801116 PMID:30962366

20. Rakesh D, Allen NB, Whittle S. Longitudinal changes in within-salience network functional connectivity mediate the relationship between childhood abuse and neglect, and mental health during adolescence. *Psychol Med*. 2021:1-13. doi:10.1017/S0033291721003135

21. Brown GW, Harris TO, Craig TKJ. Exploration of the influence of insecure attachment and parental maltreatment on the incidence and course of adult clinical depression. *Psychol Med*. 2019;49:1025-1032. doi:10.1017/S0033291718001721

22. Hughes K, Bellis MA, Hardcastle KA, et al. The effect of multiple adverse childhood experiences on health: a systematic review and meta-analysis. *Lancet Public Health*. 2017;2(8):e356-e366. doi:10.1016/s2468-2667(17)30118-4

23. Lippard ETC, Nemeroff CB. The devastating clinical consequences of child abuse and neglect: increased disease vulnerability and poor treatment response in

mood disorders. *Am J Psychiatry.* 2020;177(1):20-36. doi:10.1176/appi.ajp.2019. 19010020

24. Vachon DD, Krueger RF, Rogosch FA, Cicchetti D. Assessment of the harmful psychiatric and behavioral effects of different forms of child maltreatment. *JAMA Psychiatry.* 2015;72(11):1135. doi:10.1001/jamapsychiatry.2015.1792

25. Sheng JA, Bales NJ, Myers SA, et al. The hypothalamic-pituitary-adrenal axis: development, programming actions of hormones, and maternal-fetal interactions. *Front Behav Neurosci.* 2020;14:601939. doi:10.3389/fnbeh.2020.601939

26. Sapolsky RM, Romero LM, Munck AU. How do glucocorticoids influence stress responses? Integrating, suppressive, stimulatory and preparative actions. *Endocr Rev.* 2000;21:55-89. doi:10.1210/edrv.21

27. Smith SM, Vale WW. The role of the hypothalamic-pituitary-adrenal axis in neuroendocrine responses to stress. *Dialogues Clin Neurosci.* 2006;8(4):383-395. doi:10.31887/dcns.2006.8.4/ssmith

28. Bear MF, Connors BW, Paradiso MA. Chapter 22: Mental Illness. In: Joyce J, Francis LG, Lochhaas T, eds. *Neuroscience: Exploring the Brain.* 4th edition. Wolters Kluwer; 2016:751-780.

29. Tafet GE, Nemeroff CB. Pharmacological treatment of anxiety disorders: the role of the HPA axis. *Front Psychiatry.* 2020;11:443. doi:10.3389/fpsyt.2020.00443

30. Bunea IM, Szentágotai-Tătar A, Miu AC. Early-life adversity and cortisol response to social stress: a meta-analysis. *Transl Psychiatry.* 2017;7(12):1-8. doi:10. 1038/s41398-017-0032-3

31. Hunter AL, Minnis H, Wilson P. Altered stress responses in children exposed to early adversity: a systematic review of salivary cortisol studies. *STRESS.* 2011; 14:614-626. doi:10.3109/10253890.2011.577848

32. Marques-Feixa L, Palma-Gudiel H, Romero S, et al. Childhood maltreatment disrupts HPA-axis activity under basal and stress conditions in a dose–response relationship in children and adolescents. *Psychol Med.* 2021:1-14. doi:10.1017/ S003329172100249X

33. Turner AI, Smyth N, Hall SJ, et al. Psychological stress reactivity and future health and disease outcomes: a systematic review of prospective evidence. *Psychoneuroendocrinology.* 2020;114(104599):104599. doi:10.1016/j.psyneuen.2020. 104599

34. Basu A, McLaughlin KA, Misra S, Koenen KC. Childhood maltreatment and health impact: the examples of cardiovascular disease and type 2 diabetes mellitus in adults. *Clin Psychol (New York).* 2017;24(2):125-139. doi:10.1111/cpsp. 12191 PMID:28867878

35. American Psychiatric Association. *Diagnostic and Statistical Manual of Mental Disorders: DSM-5.* 5th ed. American Psychiatric Association; 2013.

36. Barch DM, Harms MP, Tillman R, Hawkey E, Luby JL. Early childhood depression, emotion regulation, episodic memory, and hippocampal development. *J Abnorm Psychol.* 2019;128(1):81-95. doi:10.1037/abn0000392

37. Lundy SM, Silva GE, Kaemingk KL, Goodwin JL, Quan SF. Cognitive functioning and academic performance in elementary school children with anxious/ depressed and withdrawn symptoms. *Open Pediatr Med Journal.* 2010; 4(1):1-9. doi:10.2174/1874309901004010001

38. Wagner S, Müller C, Helmreich I, Huss M, Tadić A. A meta-analysis of cognitive functions in children and adolescents with major depressive disorder. *Eur Child Adolesc Psychiatry.* 2015;24(1):5-19. doi:10.1007/s00787-014-0559-2

39. Chandler CE, Austin AE, Shanahan ME. Association of housing stress with child maltreatment: a systematic review. *Trauma Violence Abuse.* 2022;23(2):639-659. doi:10.1177/1524838020939136

40. US Department of Health and Human Services, Administration for Children and Families, Administration on Children, Youth and Families, Children's Bureau. Child Maltreatment 2020. January 2022. https://www.acf.hhs.gov/cb/data-research/child-maltreatment

41. American Psychological Association Task Force on Socioeconomic Status. Report of the APA Task Force on Socioeconomic Status. March 2008. http://www.apa.org/pi/ses/resources/publications/social-class-curricula.pdf

42. von Stumm S, Plomin R. Socioeconomic status and the growth of intelligence from infancy through adolescence. *Intelligence.* 2015;48:30-36. doi:10.1016/j.intell.2014.10.002

43. Peverill M, Dirks MA, Narvaja T, Herts KL, Comer JS, McLaughlin KA. Socioeconomic status and child psychopathology in the United States: a meta-analysis of population based studies. *Clin Psychol Rev.* 2021;83:101933. doi:10.1016/j.cpr.2020.101933

44. Cowell RA, Cicchetti D, Rogosch FA, Toth SL. Childhood maltreatment and its effect on neurocognitive functioning: timing and chronicity matter. *Dev Psychopathol.* 2015;27(2):521-533. doi:10.1017/S0954579415000139

45. De Bellis MD, Woolley DP, Hooper SR. Neuropsychological findings in pediatric maltreatment: relationship of PTSD, dissociative symptoms, and abuse/neglect indices to neurocognitive outcomes. *Child Maltreat.* 2013;18(3):171-183. doi:10.1177/1077559513497420

46. Irigaray, TQ, Pacheco JB, Grassi-Oliveira R, et al. Child maltreatment and later cognitive functioning: a systematic review. *Psicol Reflex Crítica.* 2013;26(2):376-387. doi:10.1590/S0102-79722013000200018

47. Kavanaugh B, Holler K. Brief report: neurocognitive functioning in adolescents following childhood maltreatment and evidence for underlying planning & organizational deficits. *Child Neuropsychol.* 2015;21(6):840-848. doi:10.1080/09297049.2014.929101 PMID:24955614

48. Kavanaugh BC, Dupont-Frechette JA, Jerskey BA, Holler KA. Neurocognitive deficits in children and adolescents following maltreatment: neurodevelopmental consequences and neuropsychological implications of traumatic stress. *Appl Neuropsychol Child.* 2016;6(1):64-78. doi:10.1080/21622965.2015.1079712 PMID:27050166

49. Mothes L, Kristensen CH, Grassi-Oliveira R, Fonseca RP, de Lima Argimon II, Irigaray TQ. Childhood maltreatment and executive functions in adolescents. *Child Adolesc Ment Health.* 2015;20(1):56-62. doi:10.1111/camh.12068

50. Gould F, Clarke J, Heim C, Harvey PD, Majer M, Nemeroff CB. The effects of child abuse and neglect on cognitive functioning in adulthood. *J Psychiatr Res.* 2012; 46(4):500-506. doi:10.1016/j.jpsychires.2012.01.005

51. Dunn EC, McLaughlin KA, Slopen N, Rosand J, Smoller JW. Developmental timing of child maltreatment and symptoms of depression and suicidal ideation in young adulthood: results from the National Longitudinal Study of Adolescent Health. *Depress Anxiety.* 2013;30(10):955-964. doi:10.1002/da.22102

52. Jaffee SR. Child maltreatment and risk for psychopathology in childhood and adulthood. *Annu Rev Clin Psychol.* 2017;13:525-551. doi:10.1146/annurevclinpsy-032816-045005

53. Huang S, Trapido E, Fleming L, et al. The long-term effects of childhood maltreatment experiences on subsequent illicit drug use and drug-related problems in young adulthood. *Addict Behav.* 2011;36(1-2):95-102. doi:10.1016/j.addbeh.2010.09.001

54. Romano E, Babchishin L, Marquis R, Fréchette S. Childhood maltreatment and educational outcomes. *Trauma Violence Abuse.* 2015;16(4):418-437. doi:10.1177/1524838014537908

55. Suzuki L, Aronson J. The cultural malleability of intelligence and its impact on the racial/ethnic hierarchy. *Psychol Public Policy Law.* 2005;11(2):320-327. doi:10.1037/1076-8971.11.2.320

56. Weiss LG, Saklofske DH. Mediators of IQ test score differences across racial and ethnic groups: the case for environmental and social justice. *Pers Individ Dif.* 2020;161:109962. doi:10.1016/j.paid.2020.109962

57. Croizet JC, Dutrévis M. Socioeconomic status and intelligence: why test scores do not equal merit. *J Poverty.* 2004;8(3):91-107. doi:10.1300/j134v08n03_05

58. Lezak MD, Howieson DB, Bigler ED, Tranel D. *Neuropsychological Assessment.* 5th ed. Oxford University Press; 2012.

59. Sattler JM. Correlates of intelligence. In: *Assessment of Children: Cognitive Foundations and Applications.* 6th ed. Jerome M Sattler Publisher; 2018:257-286.

60. Kavanaugh B, Holler K, Selke G. A neuropsychological profile of childhood maltreatment within an adolescent inpatient sample. *Appl Neuropsychol Child.* 2015;4(1):9-19. doi:10.1080/21622965.2013.78996

61. Kalia V, Knauft K, Hayatbini N. Adverse childhood experiences (ACEs) associated with reduced cognitive flexibility in both college and community samples. *PLoS One.* 2021;16(12):e0260822. doi:10.1371/journal.pone.0260822

62. Navalta CP, Polcari A, Webster DM, Boghossian A, Teicher MH. Effects of childhood sexual abuse on neuropsychological and cognitive function in college women. *J Neuropsychiatry Clin Neurosci.* 2006;18(1):45-53. doi:10.1176/jnp.18.1.45

63. Noll JG, Shenk CE, Yeh MT, Ji J, Putnam FW, Trickett PK. Receptive language and educational attainment for sexually abused females. *Pediatrics.* 2010;126(3). doi:10/1542/peds.2010-0496

64. Lum JAG, Powell M, Timms L, Snow P. A meta-analysis of cross sectional studies investigating language in maltreated children. *J Speech Lang Hear Res.* 2015; 58(3):961-976. doi:10.1044/2015_JSLHR-L-14-0056

65. Veltman MW, Browne KD. Three decades of child maltreatment research: implications for the school years. *Trauma Violence Abuse.* 2001;2(3):215-239. doi:10.1177/1524838001002003002

66. Snow PC. Child maltreatment, mental health and oral language competence: inviting speech-language pathology to the prevention table. *Int J Speech Lang Pathol.* 2009;11(2):95-103. doi:10.1080/17549500802415712

Chapter 3

Clinical Manifestations of Child Maltreatment

Paul Thomas Clements, PhD, RN, ANEF, DF-IAFN, DF-AFN
Theresa Fay-Hillier, DrPH, MSN, PMHCNS-BC

Objectives

After reading this chapter, the reader will be able to:

1. *Examine the traumatic presentations and behaviors related to child maltreatment.*

2. *Identify the importance of promptly reporting suspected child maltreatment to child protective services (CPS).*

3. *Identify at least 2 protective factors for children to decrease the negative impact of children encountering maltreatment.*

Background and Significance

A child's behavior is an outward manifestation of inner stability and security, and it is a lens through which health care providers can observe the development of the child.[1] Based on the level of verbal and social repertoire, children reflect their inner thoughts and feelings via demonstrations of emotional and physical behavior. All types of abuse—*physical, emotional, sexual,* and *psychological*—are damaging to children, and they can cause long-term difficulties with behavior and mental health development. Health care providers need to be aware of, and alert to, the clinical indicators of child abuse and neglect so that appropriate interventions can be provided to improve outcomes.[1,2]

Professionals in child health, primary care, mental health, schools, social services, and law enforcement all contribute to the recognition of and response to child maltreatment. However, due to a lack of awareness of the signs of child maltreatment and processes for reporting to CPS agencies, as well as a perception that reporting might do more harm than good, instances of suspected child maltreatment are underreported.[2,3]

Several widely held beliefs about child abuse and neglect may be incorrect. For example, some suggest that sexual abuse is worse than physical or emotional abuse; however, child sexual abuse is an infrequent event that is almost always accompanied by other types of child maltreatment.[4,5] Other assumptions are that each form of abuse has specific consequences and that the effects of abuse differ across sex and race. However, studies suggest that physical abuse, emotional abuse, and neglect are equivalent insults that affect broad psychiatric vulnerabilities.[4] Subsequently, recognition and reporting of all suspected or actual child maltreatment is critically important to promote child safety, health, and welfare through the provision of preventive, supportive, protective, and therapeutic interventions.

Child maltreatment is a public health problem that encompasses both the abuse and neglect of children by a parent or caregiver, which respectively include acts of commission and omission.[6] Neglect, more specifically, occurs when the basic needs of a child are not being met. These needs include the emotional, educational, nutritional, physical, supervisory, and medical requirements for proper development.[6,7] Neglect can result from the willful omission or disregard for the child or from a lack of ability or resources. This typically looks like a failure to meet the child's basic physical and emotional needs, including their access to adequate housing, food, clothing, education, and medical care.[8] Regardless of the reason for the neglect, the impact on the child's wellbeing can be the same.

Child physical abuse involves the intentional use of physical force that can result in physical injury. Examples include hitting, kicking, shaking, burning, or other shows of force against a child. Emotional abuse refers to behaviors that harm a child's self-worth or emotional wellbeing, such as name-calling, shaming, rejection, withholding love, and making threats.[8] According to the Child Abuse Prevention and Treatment Act (CAPTA),[9] sexual abuse is defined as:

> the employment, use, persuasion, inducement, enticement, or coercion of any child to engage in, or assist any other person to engage in, any sexually explicit conduct or simulation of such conduct for the purpose of producing a visual depiction of such conduct; or the rape, and in cases of caretaker or inter-familial relationships, statutory rape, molestation, prostitution, or other form of sexual exploitation of children, or incest with children.

SCOPE OF THE PROBLEM

Continued efforts have been made to improve the identification of injuries and neglect due to child maltreatment through the implementation of screening strategies. These strategies include the use of screening methods such as checklists or protocols to identify children who need targeted pediatric assessment. These methods are based on markers such as age and type of injury, repeated pattern of incidence, or a history inconsistent with the injury. There is low to very low evidence that the use of screening tools may result in higher numbers of false positives for suspected or actual child abuse. The risk for the limited occurrence of these potential false positives, therefore, is better than lack of identification of abuse through failure to use such tools in practice.[10] Subsequently, of ongoing concern is the annual rate of confirmed child maltreatment dramatically understating the cumulative number of children confirmed to be maltreated during childhood. Notably, in relation, the World Health Organization states that 1 in 5 women and 1 in 13 men report having been sexually abused between the ages of 0 and 17 years.[11]

The National Child Abuse and Neglect Data System (NCANDS)[12] states that in 2019, professionals submitted 68.6% of reports alleging child abuse and neglect. The term "professional" is used to indicate that the person has contact with the alleged child maltreatment victim as part of his or her job. These professionals include teachers, police officers, lawyers, and social services staff. The highest percentages of reports are from education personnel (21.0%), legal and law enforcement personnel (19.1%), and medical personnel (11.0%). CPS agencies received a national estimate of 4 400 000 total maltreatment-alleging referrals, which includes approximately 7 900 000 children. The national rate of screened-in referrals is 32.2 per 1000 children in the population. Among the 45 states that report both screened-in and screened-out referrals, 54.5% of referrals are screened-in and 45.5% are screened-out. Nonprofessionals, such as friends, neighbors, and relatives, submitted fewer than 1/5 of reports (15.7%). Unclassified sources, meaning anyone who reports as anonymous, other, or unknown, submitted the remaining reports (15.7%).[12]

BRAIN AND BEHAVIOR CORRELATES

Although omissions of care or lack of supervision for a child are typically obvious, the decision about whether these constitute neglect and justify a referral to CPS requires difficult judgments about what is societally and culturally acceptable behavior, whether the behavior is ongoing, and the risk of harm to the child. These judgments can be particularly challenging when a child lives in deprived circumstances (ie, comes from a refugee or asylum-seeking family) or when the child or the parent has a disability, mental health problems, or other chronic illnesses.[13]

Specific problems vary depending upon the nature, intensity, duration, and timing of neglect and abuse. Some children will have profound and obvious problems; others will have very subtle problems that do not seem to relate to early-life neglect. Neural Plasticity and Sensitive Periods[14] has become a study of note and recognition. Specifically, many aspects of brain development depend on experiences that occur during particular time periods; often the first few years of life. These so-called sensitive or critical periods represent vital inflection points in the course of development; such that, if specific experiences fail to occur within some narrow window of time (or the wrong experiences occur), development can go awry. This leads to the concept that plasticity "cuts both ways,"[14] meaning that if the child is exposed to good experiences, the brain benefits, but if the child is exposed to bad experiences or inadequate input, the brain may suffer. An example of a bad prenatal experience for the brain is exposure to and abuse of neurotoxins such as alcohol or drugs.

During childhood, the human brain matures, and brain-related capabilities develop in a sequential fashion. Newborns are almost fully dependent upon parents to help them regulate physiology and behavior. Under optimal conditions, parents are the buffer between young children and stress, serving as "co-regulators" of their child's behavior and physiology. Over time, children raised by such parents gradually assume these regulatory capacities for themselves and typically enter school demonstrating developmentally appropriate behavioral, emotional, and physiological regulation, thus being prepared for the tasks of learning and interacting with peers.[15] With optimal experiences, the brain develops healthy, flexible, and diverse capabilities. Disruptions in the timing, intensity, quality, or quantity of normal development, however, can adversely affect neurodevelopment and function. Traumatic experiences trigger a state of fear-related activation in abused and neglected children's brains. Chronic activation of the adaptive fear response can cause a persistent fear state that in turn causes hypervigilance, increased muscle tone, a focus on threat-related cues, anxiety, and behavioral impulsivity. These attributes are helpful during a threatening event but counterproductive once the threat has passed. The very process of proper adaptive neural response during a threat underlies the neural pathology that causes distress and pain throughout a child's life. The chronically traumatized child will develop a host of physical signs (eg, altered cardiovascular regulation) and symptoms (eg, attention, sleep, and mood problems) that make life more difficult.[16]

A strong and secure attachment bond with a primary caregiver is at the core of developing resilience and a healthy personality. This bond strengthens a child's ability to cope with stress, regulates their emotions, provides social support, and forms nurturing relationships.[17] When this type of bond exists, the world is experienced as a safe place in which to explore and develop independence, and the child finds comfort and support from his or her caregiver when under stress. When children are abused, they might display disturbed forms of attachment and abnormal patterns of emotional response toward their caregivers.[17,18]

Childhood maltreatment is a stressor that can lead to the development of behavior problems, and it affects brain structure and function. Neuropsychological studies suggest an association between child abuse and deficits in IQ, memory, working memory, attention, response inhibition, and emotion discrimination. Structural neuroimaging studies provide evidence for deficits in brain volume, gray and white matter of several regions, dorsolateral and ventromedial prefrontal cortex, hippocampus, amygdala, and corpus callosum.[18,19] Early childhood abuse has many behavioral consequences, of which most prominently is the internalizing of behavioral problems such as limited stress tolerance, anxiety, affective instability, depression, suicidality, post-traumatic stress disorder, dissociative disturbances, and hallucinatory phenomena. However, there are also externalizing behavioral symptoms such as poor impulse control, episodic aggression, substance abuse, ADHD, and conduct disorder.[20,21]

Studies of adverse childhood experiences (ACEs), such as maltreatment, have reported mental, physical, behavioral, and social consequences well into adulthood. As an example, children who have experienced abuse or neglect are more likely to have depression and diabetes as adults, to have difficulties with relationships, to struggle with substance abuse, and to be involved in violence and criminal behavior.[22]

When monitored into adolescence and adulthood, deficiencies in reading ability and academic performance have been documented in children who were physically abused. Several prospective studies have established that poor school performance (eg, poor grades, low scores on standardized achievement tests, grade retention, placement in special education) is often an outcome of childhood abuse and neglect.[14] Furthermore, there is fairly consistent evidence that child maltreatment often has negative consequences for cognitive functioning and academic performance, beginning in early childhood and extending into adulthood. These consequences are not exclusively found in physically abused children; they have been reported in neglected children as well.[14,16,17]

Furthermore, children model adult behavior; therefore, maltreated children who learn that abusive behavior is the "right" way to interact with others tend to have problems in later social situations. For example, children who have been sexually abused are at risk of being further victimized or perpetrating abuse against younger children.[19]

The lifelong outcomes related to early maltreatment experiences are thought to have pervasive effects of toxic stress on the brain and body.[23,24] When children feel threatened, their bodies prepare to respond by increasing their heart rate, blood pressure, and stress hormones (eg, cortisol). When a child's stress response systems are activated within an environment of supportive parent or caregiver relationships, these physiological effects are buffered and brought back down to baseline. The result is the development of healthy stress response systems, which is an important part of healthy child development. However, if the stress response is extreme, long-lasting, and buffering relationships are unavailable to the child, the result can be damaged, weakened systems and brain architecture with lifelong repercussions.[25]

In light of the significant potential for both short-term and long-term behavioral, educational, and health implications of stress for child victims of trauma and violence, it is important to distinguish the 3 kinds of responses to stress: *positive*, *tolerable*, and *toxic*. As described below, these 3 terms refer to the stress response systems' effects on the body, not to the stressful event or experience itself[25]:

— *Positive stress response* is a normal and essential part of healthy development, characterized by brief increases in heart rate and mild elevations in hormone levels. Some situations that might trigger a positive stress response are the first day with a new caregiver or receiving an injected immunization.

— *Tolerable stress response* activates the body's alert systems to a greater degree because of more severe, longer-lasting difficulties such as the loss of a loved one, a natural disaster, or a frightening injury. If the activation is time-limited and buffered by relationships with adults who help the child adapt, the brain and other organs recover from what might otherwise be damaging effects.

— *Toxic stress response* can occur when a child experiences strong, frequent, or prolonged adversity (eg, physical or emotional abuse, chronic neglect, caregiver substance abuse or mental illness, exposure to violence, the accumulated burdens of family economic hardship) without adequate adult support. This kind of prolonged activation of the stress response systems can disrupt the development of brain architecture and other organ systems as well as increase the risk for stress-related disease and cognitive impairment well into the adult years.

RISK AND PROTECTIVE FACTORS

Over the years, many risk factors for different forms of child maltreatment have been identified in large bodies of research. Multiple studies have shown that the cumulation of risk factors rather than the presence of a single risk factor is predictive of future child maltreatment. For example, one study noted that since parental risk factors play an important role in the (re)occurrence of child maltreatment, they should therefore be the primary focus when preventing child maltreatment.[26] Subsequently, the researchers recommended that clinicians should assess for the following risk factors in an interrelated approach toward prevention and assessment of child abuse:

— Caregiver has a history of abusing a child

— Caregiver has a psychiatric disorder

— Caregiver has an addiction

— Caregiver has a mental disability

— Caregiver is physically absent

— Caregiver is emotionally absent

— Caregiver was maltreated as a child

— Caregiver has been violent before

— Caregiver(s) have a problematic relationship

— There is family conflict

— A history of domestic violence

— Parental stress about financial problems

— Social isolation of the family

To further deal with the potential multi-risk level of recognizing emotional trauma related to child maltreatment, it has been argued that children should be screened for trauma exposure and symptoms at all childcare visits by asking, "Since the last time I saw you, has anything really scary or upsetting happened to you or your family?"[1] By directly addressing the child, practitioners can better assess for possible adverse experiences. Because maltreatment causes stress that is associated with disruption in early brain development as well as development of the nervous and immune systems, maltreated children are at an increased risk for behavioral, physical, and mental health problems.

Simultaneous to assessing for risks, the clinician should employ an assets-based approach, keeping in mind that protective factors can mitigate the negative impact of ACEs. Sege & Browne[27] identified Health Outcomes from Positive Experiences (HOPE) that can increase the potential of favorable health outcomes for children who have encountered ACEs. For example, children's optimism, high self-esteem, intelligence, creativity, humor, and independence can enhance their coping skills in the face of adversity. The acceptance of peers and positive influences such as teachers, mentors, and role models can provide a foundation for channeling and dissipating stressful and traumatic situations. The family's access to social supports, neighborhood stability, safe schools, and adequate health care are of note for assessment, as these provide necessary facets for timely and adaptive intrapsychic growth and development.[28,29]

Clinicians should help caregivers identify the protective factors that are going to be crucial during the rigorous path towards healing. Providers should further remind caregivers that seeking respite care can be immensely beneficial (and is not a sign of failure) and that they should also rely on friends, family, and community resources. Many communities have support groups for families confronting the impact of child maltreatment. In sum, the child's experience of love, acceptance, positive guidance, and protection coming from a caring adult encourages trust that they will be provided with what they need to thrive. Parents' or caregivers' respectful communication and listening, consistent rules and expectations, and safe opportunities that promote independence significantly facilitate this environment and process. Instilling a pattern of adaptive coping in the face of adversity, whether expected or sudden, is crucial to the child's development. This development is enhanced when parents or caregivers have a social network of emotionally supportive friends, family, and neighbors who can meet their own basic needs for food, clothing, housing, and transportation and know how to access essential services such as childcare, health care, and mental health services.[19,24,28]

PROVIDING SUPPORT FOR MALTREATED CHILDREN

Bruce Perry,[29] a pioneer in the field of the effects of trauma and neglect on children, notes several primary factors inherent to successful care and support. Foundational to this fertile environment for adaptation and growth are responsive, nurturing adults (eg, parents, teachers, and other caregivers). Children need to be nurtured via holding, rocking, and cuddling. However, there is a need for simultaneous awareness that for many children, touch has been associated with pain, torture, or sexual abuse. It is imperative for clinicians to observe how a child responds to nurturing and act accordingly. In many ways, these interactions provide experiences that should have taken place during infancy.[29,30]

Many abused and neglected children do not know how to interact with other people, as they are often emotionally and socially delayed. Therefore, it is important to interact with children at their perceived emotional age. Maltreated children will often use very primitive, immature, and bizarre soothing behaviors. They may bite themselves, head bang, rock, chant, scratch, or cut themselves, and these symptoms will increase during times of distress or threat.[5,31] When they are frustrated or fearful, they will regress, and as much as one may want the children to "act their age," they simply cannot. If they are tearful, frustrated, or overwhelmed (eg, demonstrating developmental emotionality of age 2), a practitioner should use soothing nonverbal interactions.[27,28]

Clinicians should be consistent, predictable, and repetitive. Maltreated children with attachment issues are very sensitive to new situations. Social events (eg, parties, sleepovers, trips) can overwhelm them, even if the events are a pleasant experience. Efforts to make life consistent, predictable, and repetitive are very important. When children feel safe, they can benefit from nurturing and enriching experiences. Additionally, clinicians should model and teach appropriate social behaviors. To teach them, providers should model appropriate behaviors and narrate for the child what they are doing and why (ie, "I am going to the sink to wash my hands before dinner because..." or "I take the soap and put it on my hands like this....").[31]

Maltreated children can also have problems modulating physical contact. Child maltreatment is associated with disruptions in physiological arousal, emotion regulation, and defensive responses to cues of threat and distress, as well as increased risk for callous unemotional traits and externalizing behavior.[32,33] Children who have experienced maltreatment, for example, do not know when to hug, how close to stand, when to make or break eye contact, or at what times they can wipe their nose, touch their genitals, or do grooming and daily hygiene tasks. A provider should try not to lecture the child about "appropriate behavior," and should instead gently suggest how they can interact differently with adults and children (eg, "Why don't you sit over here?"). Clinicians should also make lessons clear using as few words as possible and explain them in a way that will not make the child feel bad or guilty. Providers can even coach maltreated children as they play with other children using play-by-play (eg, "Well, when you take that from someone, they probably feel pretty upset. So, if you want them to have fun when you play this game, then you should try…."). Over time, success with other children will make the child less socially awkward and aggressive.[32,33]

Clinicians should strive to understand the behaviors of maltreated children before punishing them. More specifically, it is important for providers to be mindful as to whether they are handing down *punishment* or whether they are providing *constructive consequences*.[34] Children with trauma are vulnerable when they are disciplined—even more so when their trauma is extensive—so discipline should be administered carefully. Clinicians should try to be as gentle as possible while still holding reasonable and safe guidelines. Before setting limits or punishing, it is important for the provider to be able to clearly state the expectations. Additionally, while providers always want to address the emotions first before problem solving/advice/consequences, it is imperative to remember that children with trauma can have a hard time identifying emotions and dealing with emotional dysregulation, so it is best to be mindful. In this same vein, to avoid undermining any proactive interventions, clinicians must simultaneously monitor their own emotions.[24,28,30]

It is imperative for providers to actively listen to and talk *with* children (versus talking *at* them). When providers are quiet and interactive, children will often begin to share their experiences through storytelling and demonstrating events (ie, "show and tell" opportunities). Providers should create an environment in which children feel relaxed and know that they are not being rushed into the next steps of treatment. This subsequently becomes a strategic opportunity to teach children about their feelings. It is helpful to use the following principles: (1) all feelings (eg, sad, glad, mad) are okay to feel; (2) children should know healthy ways to act out their emotions; (3) teach empathy by highlighting that other people have emotions too, and then show those feelings (eg, "How do you think Bobby feels when you push him?"), and (4) ask children how they are feeling when it is clear that they are demonstrating an emotion.[27,29,35-37]

When developing a treatment plan, providers should ensure that they have realistic expectations (particularly recognizing the developmental level of the child versus the expected behaviors based on the age of the child) and keep in mind that abused and neglected children have a lot to overcome. Although it is not possible to accurately predict potential, providers do know how to measure a child's emotional, behavioral, social, and physical strengths and weaknesses. Skilled clinicians can help to define a child's skill areas and areas where progress will be slower.[22] It is also important for both clinicians and providers to be patient with a traumatized child's progress and with themselves, as the process may be slow and frustrating. Many adults may feel inadequate because all the support, time, and effort that they exert on a child's behalf may not seem to work. However, research and history show that it does work; it just takes time.[1,22,29] Caring for maltreated children can be exhausting and demoralizing. Clinicians and caregivers cannot provide the consistent, predictable, enriching, and nurturing care that these children need if they themselves are depleted; both rest and support are crucial.[38]

SUMMARY
A growing number of experts are formally categorizing childhood trauma as a public health crisis.[39-41] Although trauma manifests differently with each child developmentally and behaviorally, there are some commonalities, and noticing the signs can

help a clinician determine the best ways to help. A child's experiences during their formative years are especially meaningful, as they lay the foundation for the rest of a child's life. Unresolved or unprocessed trauma can have significant consequences for children, leaving a negative impact that lasts well into their adult life.[27,41] Children must receive the help they need to resolve sources of conflict, prevent long-term suffering, and begin healing. When upsetting things happen to a child, their parents, teachers, and other caregivers must try to help them work through their distress in a healthy way. How a child responds following a traumatic event will differ based on both their developmental stage and chronological age. It is essential to know the signs of trauma in children, as the impact of unresolved trauma can last for years.

KEY POINTS

1. While the adaptive fear response is crucial in human development, chronic activation can cause a persistent fear state that in turn causes hypervigilance, increased muscle tone, a focus on threat-related cues, anxiety, and behavioral impulsivity.

2. Prompt reporting of suspected child maltreatment to CPS is critical to promoting child safety through identified necessary interventions.

3. A child's experience of love, acceptance, positive guidance, and protection from a caring, respectful adult caregiver who is able to listen and communicate effectively encourages trust that the child will be provided with what they need to thrive.

REFERENCES

1. Al Odhayani A, Watson WJ, Watson L. Behavioural consequences of child abuse. *Can Fam Physician*. 2013;59(8):831-836.

2. Pekarsky AR. Overview of child maltreatment (child abuse). 2020. https://www.merckmanuals.com/professional/pediatrics/child-maltreatment/overview-of-child-maltreatment

3. LeCroy WL, Milligan-LeCroy S. Public perceptions of child maltreatment: a national convenience sample. *Child Youth Serv Rev*. 2020:119. doi:10.1016/j.childyouth.2020.105677

4. Lippard ETC, Nemeroff CB. The devastating clinical consequences of child abuse and neglect: increase disease vulnerability and poor treatment response in mood disorder. *Am J Psych*. 2019;77(1)20-36. doi:10.1176/appi.ajp.2019.19010020

5. US Department of Health and Human Services. What is child abuse and neglect? Recognizing the signs and symptoms. Child Welfare Information Gateway. 2019. https://www.childwelfare.gov/pubpdfs/whatiscan.pdf

6. Jackson AM, Kissoon N, Greene C. Aspects of abuse: recognizing and responding to child maltreatment. *Curr Probl Pediatr Adolesc Health Care*. 2015;45(3):58-70. doi:10.1016/j.cppeds.2015.02.001

7. Definitions of child abuse and neglect. Child Welfare Information Gateway. 2019. https://www.childwelfare.gov/pubpdfs/define.pdf

8. Fast facts: preventing child abuse & neglect. Centers for Disease Control and Prevention. 2021. https://www.cdc.gov/violenceprevention/childabuseandneglect/fastfact.html

9. Child Abuse Prevention and Treatment and Adoption Reform (CAPTA): Definitions. 42 USCA §5106g(a)(4) (2019). https://www.govinfo.gov/app/details/USCODE-2010-title42/USCODE-2010-title42-chap67-subchapI-sec5106g

10. McTavish JR, Gonzalez A, Santesso N, et al. Identifying children exposed to maltreatment: a systematic review update. *BMC Pediatr*. 2020;20;113. doi:10.1186/s12887-020-2015-4

11. Child maltreatment; key facts. World Health Organization. 2020. https://www. who.int/news-room/fact-sheets/detail/child-maltreatment#:~:text=Key%20 facts%20Nearly%203%20in%204%20children%20-,sexually%20abused%20 as%20a%20child%20aged%200-17%20years

12. Child maltreatment 2019. US Department of Health and Human Services; Administration for Children and Families; Administration on Children, Youth and Families; Children's Bureau. 2021. www.acf.hhs.gov/cb/research-data-technology/ statistics-research/child-maltreatment

13. Committee on Child Maltreatment Research, Policy, and Practice for the Next Decade: Phase II; Board on Children, Youth, and Families; Committee on Law and Justice; Institute of Medicine; National Research Council; Petersen AC, Joseph J, Feit M, eds. *New Directions in Child Abuse and Neglect Research.* National Academies Press; 2014. https://www.ncbi.nlm.nih.gov/books/ NBK195987/

14. White EJ, Hutka SA, Williams LJ, Moreno S. Learning, neural plasticity, and sensitive periods: implications for language acquisition, music training, and transfer across the lifespan. *Front Sys Neurosci.* 2013;7:90. doi:10.3389/fnsys.2013.00090

15. Nelson CA 3rd, Zeanah CH, Fox NA. How early experience shapes human development: the case of psychosocial deprivation. *Neural Plast.* 2019;2019: 1676285. doi:10.1155/2019/1676285

16. Owlsby D. What's the impact of abuse and neglect on the developing brain? Relavate Counseling Ministry. 2018. https://www.relavate.org/babies/2018/7/15/ the-impact-of-abuse-and-neglect-on-the-developing-grain

17. Key concepts: resilience. Harvard University; Center on the Developing Child. 2022. https://developingchild.harvard.edu/science/key-concepts/resilience/

18. Erozkan A. The link between types of attachment and childhood trauma. *Univers J Educ Res.* 2016;4(5):1071-1079. doi:10.13189/ujer.2016.040517

19. Nelson CA 3rd, Bhutta ZA, Harris NB, Danese A, Samara M. Adversity in childhood is linked to mental and physical health throughout life. *BMJ.* 2020; 371:3048. doi:10.1136/bmj.m3048

20. Hart H, Rubia K. Neuroimaging of child abuse: a critical review. *Front Hum Neurosci.* 2012;6:52. doi:10.3389/fnhum.2012.00052

21. Substance Abuse and Mental Health Services Administration Center for Behavioral Health Statistics and Quality. DSM-5 changes: implications for child serious emotional disturbance. 2016. https://www.samhsa.gov/data/sites/default/ files/NSDUH-DSM5ImpactChildSED-2016.pdf

22. Recognizing and treating child traumatic stress. Substance Abuse and Mental Health Services Administration. 2022. https://www.samhsa.gov/child-trauma/ recognizing-and-treating-child-traumatic-stress

23. Fast facts: prevention adverse childhood experiences. Centers for Disease Control and Prevention. 2022. https://www.cdc.gov/violenceprevention/aces/fastfact.html

24. Education in crisis and conflict. Key concepts on child development: toxic stress. USAID. 2022. https://www.edu-links.org/resources/key-concepts-child-development-toxic-stress

25. Toxic stress. Center on the Developing Child, Harvard University. 2023. https:// developingchild.harvard.edu/science/key-concepts/toxic-stress/

26. Annemiek V, van der Put C, Geert Jan JM, Stams JK, Assink M. Exploring the interrelatedness of risk factors for child maltreatment: a network approach. *Child Abuse Negl.* 2020;107:104622. doi:10.1016/j.chiabu.2020.104622

27. Sege RD, Browne CH. Responding to ACEs with HOPE: health outcomes from positive experiences. *Acad Pediatr.* 2017;17(7S):S79-S85. doi:10.1016/j.acap.2017.03.007

28. Complete guide to managing behavior problems. Child Mind Institute. 2023. https://childmind.org/guide/parents-guide-to-problem-behavior/

29. Perry BD. Supporting maltreated children: countering the effects of neglect and abuse. North American Council on Adopted Children. 2022. https://nacac.org/resource/supporting-maltreated-children/

30. Divecha D. Hitting children leads to trauma, not better behavior. Developmental Science. February 10, 2022. https://www.developmentalscience.com/blog/2022/2/10/hitting-children-leads-to-trauma-not-better-behavior

31. Attachment disorders in children: causes, symptoms, and treatment. HelpGuide. 2022. https://www.helpguide.org/articles/parenting-family/attachment-issues-and-reactive-attachment-disorders.htm

32. Oshri A, Carlson M, Duprey E, Liu S, Huffman L, Kogan S. Child abuse and neglect, callous-unemotional traits, and substance use problems: the moderating role of stress response reactivity. *J Child Adolesc Trauma.* 2020;13:389-398. doi:10.1007/s40653-019-00291-z

33. Dackis M, Rogosch F, Cicchetti D. Child maltreatment, callous–unemotional traits, and defensive responding in high-risk children: an investigation of emotion-modulated startle response. *Dev Psychopathol.* 2015;27(4pt2):1527-1545. doi:10.1017/S0954579415000929

34. Pincus D. Punishments vs. consequences: which are you using? 2022. https://www.empoweringparents.com/article/punishments-vs-consequences-which-are-you-using/

35. Tantrum B. 10 tips for disciplining traumatized children. Northwest Trauma Counseling. http://www.nwtraumacounseling.org/family-resources/10-tips-for-disciplining-a-traumatized-child

36. Managing your emotional reactions. The Nemours Foundation. 2022. https://kidshealth.org/en/teens/emotional-reactions.html

37. Trauma informed care in behavioral health services. Substance Abuse and Mental Health Services Administration. 2014. https://store.samhsa.gov/sites/default/files/d7/priv/sma14-4816.pdf

38. Protective factors to promote well-being and prevent child abuse & neglect. Child Welfare Information Gateway. 2020. https://www.childwelfare.gov/topics/preventing/promoting/protectfactors/

39. Understanding child trauma. Substance Abuse and Mental Health Services Administration. 2023. https://www.samhsa.gov/child-trauma/understanding-child-trauma

40. Child abuse and neglect prevention. Centers for Disease Control and Prevention. 2022. https://www.cdc.gov/violenceprevention/childabuseandneglect/index.html

41. About the CDC-Kaiser Permanente ACE study. Centers for Disease Control and Prevention. 2021. https://www.cdc.gov/violenceprevention/aces/about.html

Section II

MENTAL HEALTH ASSESSMENT

CHILD MALTREATMENT IN THE POST-PANDEMIC ERA

Paul Thomas Clements, PhD, RN, ANEF, DF-IAFN, DF-AFN

Mitzy D. Flores, PhDc, MSN, RN, AHN-BC, CHSE, COI, Caritas Coach©,
    Introspective Hypnosis Practitioner

OBJECTIVES

After reading this chapter, the reader will be able to:

1. *Describe the evolution and ongoing changes in child maltreatment in the Post-Pandemic Era.*

2. *Examine the role of risk and protective factors in the Post-Pandemic Era.*

3. *Identify the foundational importance of maintaining social connections toward adaptive mental health in children.*

BACKGROUND AND SIGNIFICANCE

As we write this chapter, the day in which COVID-19 has been declared no longer a pandemic, both nationally[1] and globally,[2] has finally arrived. At this point, medical projections indicate that outbreaks only have as much potential as do cases of influenza, and that COVID-19 vaccines will likely become annual like flu shots. Specifically, White House officials anticipate a schedule similar to that of the annual influenza vaccine, with annual updated COVID-19 shots matched to the currently circulating strains.[3] Although we acknowledge that COVID-19 will become a permanent, albeit now less acute, medical situation in the global society, we are simultaneously hoping that the impact it has had on the worsening of prevalence and severity of child maltreatment will eventually lessen. However, we still posit that this chapter remains necessary as a preface to the chapters that follow, believing it relevant to the significant amount of violence and abuse that occurred during this unanticipated period in history–specifically, the historically dubbed "pandemic." Even if the direct social, emotional, and economic impacts of COVID-19 are no longer actively driving factors to the correlates of child maltreatment, we believe it is important to cast light on the interface of this unique (and unanticipated) public health catastrophe and the impact of the unique Adverse Childhood Experiences (ACEs)[4] that occurred during that discrete period of time on the subsequent navigation of childhood growth and development.

In 2020, the American Psychiatric Association issued a statement indicating that COVID-19 may increase domestic violence and child abuse,[5] specifically stating:

> As the nation grapples with the spread of COVID-19, Americans are being told to go home and stay there, for their safety and everyone else's. But for victims and survivors of domestic violence, including children exposed to it, being home may not be a safe option—and the unprecedented stress of the pandemic could breed unsafety in homes where violence may not have been an issue before.

Further, during this time, shelters were closing or under-resourced, emergency rooms were full, and people did not want to go out in public due to the risk of COVID-19.

The things people were once instructed to readily use in their safety plan were no longer available, leaving victims trapped in an escalating cycle of tension, power, and control. Unfortunately, even with the eventual public health efforts to control the spread of COVID-19, this ultimately led to an ongoing limited or restricted availability of resources for children being exposed to, or as direct recipients of, violence, neglect, and other forms of maltreatment.

We now find ourselves in the "post-pandemic" era—where child abuse and neglect remain common. There were 4 000 000 child maltreatment referral reports received in 2021 involving 7 200 000 children, representing 90.6% of victims, being maltreated by one or both parents. Ultimately, an estimated 1820 of those children died from abuse and neglect.[6] In this new era, the nation's health care (and mental health care) turns toward an expanded awareness of the interface and impact of social determinants of health on child maltreatment.[7,8] Experiencing poverty can place a lot of stress on families, potentially increasing the risk for child abuse and neglect. Rates of child abuse and neglect are 5 times higher for children in families with low socioeconomic status compared to children in families with higher socioeconomic status.[9] Additionally, child maltreatment is costly. Peterson et al[10] estimated an increase in the per victim lifetime economic burden of child maltreatment from $210 012 to $830 928 per child victim. Furthermore, the overall financial cost of child abuse and neglect in the United States is estimated at $585 billion.[6]

RISK AND PROTECTIVE FACTORS IN THE POST-PANDEMIC ERA

Young children experience the world by proxy through their relationships with parents and other caregivers. Safe, stable, nurturing relationships and environments are essential to preventing child abuse and neglect. The American Psychological Association notes social factors that put individuals at a higher risk for violence, which include reduced access to resources, increased stress due to job loss or strained finances, and disconnection from social support systems; furthermore, within the scope of COVID-19, when these factors occur, it may lead to circumstances that foster violence.[5] Parental depression, for example, has been noted to be a significant predictor of harsh parenting and has been emphasized in etiological models as a key risk factor for child maltreatment.[11] Consequently, the odds of being psychologically maltreated and physically abused during COVID-19 were noted to be 112 and 20 times higher, respectively, among children that were maltreated in the year prior to the pandemic.[12] Additionally, children with special education, intellectual, or developmental needs are also at risk, as they may become agitated because of the disruption to their daily routines, thereby increasing the tension at home, potentially leading to physical abuse and neglect.[5,13]

Risk factors are characteristics that may increase the likelihood of experiencing or perpetrating child abuse and neglect, but they may or may not be direct causes. A combination of individual, relational, community, and societal factors contribute to the risk of child abuse and neglect[14] (see **Table 4-1**). Although children are *never* responsible for the harm inflicted upon them, certain factors have been found to increase their risk of being abused or neglected. The Centers for Disease Control and Prevention (CDC) has provided a public access educational video, "Moving Forward,"[15] to help viewers learn more about how to increase the factors that protect people from violence and reduce the factors that put people at risk. It is informative for both clinicians and the general public.

Research to date suggests that childhood trauma causes permanent damage to key brain structures involved in emotion, memory, and regulation, thereby affecting interpersonal behavior and awareness (eg, the ability to empathize).[16] Violence in the home can also lead to adverse health and mental health outcomes, including a higher risk of chronic disease, depression, post-traumatic stress disorder, and risky sexual and substance use behaviors.[16-18] Repeated exposure to traumatic experiences changes the responsiveness in the hypothalamus-pituitary-adrenal (HPA) axis with lasting consequences in the developing brain structures, such as the hippocampus and amygdala. These physiological changes are thought to cause a range of mental disorders, which are associated with poor affect regulation, anxiety, depression, and potential for substance misuse.[19-21]

Table 4-1. Risk Factors for Victimization and Offender Behavior[14]	
SCALE	RISK FACTORS
Individual Risk Factors	— Children younger than 4 years of age
	— Children with special needs that may increase caregiver burden (eg, disabilities, mental health issues, chronic physical illnesses)
Family Risk Factors	— Families that have family members in jail or prison
	— Families that are isolated from and not connected to other people (eg, extended family, friends, neighbors)
	— Family violence, including relationship violence
	— Families with high conflict and negative communication styles
Community Risk Factors	— Communities with high rates of violence and crime
	— Communities with high rates of poverty and limited educational and economic opportunities
	— Communities with high unemployment rates
	— Communities with easy access to drugs and alcohol
	— Communities where neighbors do not know or look out for each other and there is low community involvement among residents
	— Communities with few community activities for young people
	— Communities with unstable housing and where residents move frequently
	— Communities where families frequently experience food insecurity
Risk Factors for Perpetration	— Caregivers with drug or alcohol issues
	— Caregivers with mental health issues, including depression
	— Caregivers who do not understand children's needs or development
	— Caregivers who were abused or neglected as children
	— Caregivers who are young, single parents, or parents with many children
	— Caregivers with low education or income
	— Caregivers experiencing high levels of parenting stress and economic stress
	— Caregivers who use spanking and other forms of corporal punishment for discipline
	— Caregivers in the home who are not a biological parent
	— Caregivers with attitudes accepting of or justifying violence or aggression

PROTECTIVE AND COMPENSATORY FACTORS IN THE POST-PANDEMIC ERA

Protective and compensatory factors (otherwise referred to as positive and adverse childhood experiences [PACEs] or Positive Childhood Experiences)[22-24] are conditions or attributes of individuals, families, communities, and larger society that mitigate risk and promote the healthy development and wellbeing of children, adolescents, and families. Protective factors help ensure that children and adolescents are functioning well at home, in school, at work, and in the community. There are 5 key protective factors that are generally acknowledged to serve as buffers and help parents find resources, support, and coping strategies that allow them to parent effectively, even under stress. These are[24]:

— *Parental Resilience.* Managing stress and functioning well when faced with challenges, adversity, and trauma

— *Social Connections.* Positive relationships that provide emotional, informational, instrumental, and spiritual support

— *Knowledge of Parenting and Child Development.* Understanding child development and parenting strategies that support physical, cognitive, language, social, and emotional development

— *Concrete Supports in Time of Need.* Access to concrete supports and services that address a family's needs and help minimize stress caused by challenges

— *Social and Emotional Competence in Children.* Family and child interactions that help children develop the ability to communicate clearly, recognize and regulate their emotions, and establish and maintain relationships

Providers should be actively assessing for and promoting these attributes when interacting with families who are at risk for abuse and maltreatment, particularly since there is now no longer limited access to supportive mental health treatment and referral due to mandatory lockdowns and quarantine orders.

COMMUNICATION

Even before COVID-19, children's mental health was a public health concern, and levels of anxiety were on the rise. COVID-19 resulted in additional stress, fear, and worry for many families. Worries about sickness, finances, and isolation, coping with grief from loss, and having less outside help often resulted in escalating tensions and episodic or patterned violence.[25-27] Just as COVID-19 affected the social lives of adults, it also affected the social lives of young children. Early on in life, children learn how to interact with other people, including their peers. They build their communication, language, speech, and social skills by watching and listening to their peers, older children, their parents, and other adults in their lives. Since COVID-19 began, young children did not have access to many natural opportunities to interact with others and develop these essential skills. For those children living in chaotic households within which violence and other traumatic events occurred, caregivers are consistently faced with the challenges of explaining the complexities of these situations in a manner that is relatable to young minds. It is recommended that in these conversations, clinicians and caregivers should begin by creating an atmosphere that promotes support and openness—allowing children to inquire about the violence and traumatic events yet responding with openness and gentleness.

Since there have not been as many opportunities to interact with family and other age-equivalent friends, children have not had as much opportunity to spend time with people other than their parents or siblings. While parents are the most important communication partner for young children, especially in the early years, it is still important for children to communicate with unfamiliar listeners.[28] Providers should use words and concepts the child can comprehend, and which are appropriate for their developmental stage. Additionally, they should have sources prepared so that children can be guided to explore acceptable data if they would like more information. When these conversations develop, validation of the child's emotional responses is crucial. Providers should support the child by letting them know that they believe they had great questions and feedback. Children tend to personalize situations and may worry a great deal about certain circumstances and how they could affect their loved ones and friends. Therefore, providers must be patient, be prepared to repeat information, and reassure the child, as they may require extra support to ease their anxieties and worries. Signs that a child may need additional professional support by a mental health practitioner include constant preoccupation about how the violence can affect them and their family, sleep disturbances, constant thoughts of illness or death, and not wanting to attend social gatherings or school due to fear.[29,30]

MAINTAINING SOCIAL CONNECTIONS

For children who have returned to school, changes to the space and to routines may have made everything look and feel different. Being around masked faces for an extended period may have added to a child's feelings of uncertainty, because facial expressions help communicate feelings and provide assurance, and wearing masks makes this difficult. In this post-pandemic era, as children look to their parents for signs of safety, parents may need to put more effort into expressing confidence and security with words and body language in addition to facial expressions.[31] This is particularly important for young children who are not yet able to talk about feelings. Children are generally flexible and can adapt, but strategies that protect children's health may make transitions to new situations and new people harder. According to Harvard University's Center on the Developing Child,[32] it is recommended that caregivers practice "serve and return," which is a technique of back-and-forth inter-action. These kinds of interactions help with brain development and resilience as well as reduce the effects of ongoing stress. Ways to promote responsive relationships between child and caregiver may include the incorporation of electronics, such as video chatting or phone calls. Caregivers can also encourage writing emails or letters to family and friends.

Furthermore, new activities should be implemented into the family's routines. Activi-ties can include family game times, which can be anything from board games to cook-ing to dancing to playing together as a family unit. Other social activities can include physical fitness tasks like going out for walks, bike riding, or doing yoga together, which promote physical and mental wellbeing. Finally, caregivers should make plans for all these social connections and activities. Making plans helps the child visualize the immediate future. Additionally, children will be able to watch as adults promote problem solving responses during a crisis, and this may be helpful in reassuring the child that they are supported and safe.

CONCLUSION

COVID-19 had a devastating impact across the world, and efforts to re-equilibrate will take both time and concerted efforts on the parts of clinicians and caregivers. Additionally, the effects of abuse and trauma from prolonged and isolated periods of time with abusers and traumatic situations will continue to have an impact.[33-35] COVID-19 also exposed children to increased risks of violence, including maltreatment, gender-based violence, and sexual exploitation, as they were disconnected from many community resources and support systems. Research shows that increased stress levels among parents is often a major predictor of physical abuse and neglect of children. Stressed parents may be more likely to respond to their children's anxious behaviors or demands in aggressive or abusive ways. The home may not be safe for many families who experience domestic violence, which may include both intimate partners and children. COVID-19 has contributed toward widespread uncertainty and panic; therefore, during this time of readjustment to post-pandemic conditions, clinicians must ensure that they are still actively screening patients for intimate partner violence and child abuse.

KEY POINTS

1. COVID-19 has contributed to widespread uncertainty and tensions; therefore, during the post-pandemic era, health care practitioners must ensure that they are screening patients for intimate partner violence and child abuse.

2. COVID-19 has directly impacted social factors that put individuals at a higher risk for violence, which include increased stress due to job loss or strained finances, losses that have altered family structure, and disconnection from social support systems.

3. Caregivers of children are consistently faced with the challenges of explaining the complexities of violence and trauma in a manner that is relatable to young minds. Keeping the conversation simple is key.

ADDITIONAL RESOURCES (Table 4-2)

Table 4-2. Addressing Intimate Partner Violence and Child Maltreatment Concerns	
ORGANIZATION	CONTACT INFORMATION
SAMHSA's National Helpline (Substance Abuse and Mental Health Services Administration)	1-800-662-HELP (4357)
National Child Abuse Hotline	1-800-4-A-CHILD (800-422-4453)
National Domestic Violence Hotline	1-800-799-SAFE (7233)
Military One Source: Preventing Abuse and Neglect	1-800-342-9647
StrongHearts Native Helpline	1-844-762-8483
National Suicide Prevention Lifeline	1-800-273-8255

If this is an emergency, call 911. To report suspected child maltreatment, contact a county department of Social Services.

REFERENCES

1. End of the federal COVID-19 Public Health Emergency (PHE) declaration. Centers for Disease Control and Prevention. May 5, 2023. https://www.cdc.gov/coronavirus/2019-ncov/your-health/end-of-phe.html#:~:text=The%20federal%20COVID%2D19%20PHE,share%20certain%20data%20will%20change

2. WHO Chief declares end to COVID-19 as a global health emergency. United Nations. May 5, 2023. https://news.un.org/en/story/2023/05/1136367#:~:text=WHO%20chief%20declares%20end%20to%20COVID%2D19%20as%20a%20global%20health%20emergency,-5%20May%202023&text=The%20head%20of%20the%20UN,no%20longer%20a%20global%20threat

3. Bendix A. Covid vaccines will likely become annual like flu shots, White House officials say. NBC News. September 6, 2022. Accessed September 6,

2022. https://www.nbcnews.com/health/health-news/covid-vaccines-likely-annu-al-like-flu-shots-rcna46456#

4. Adverse Childhood Experiences (ACEs). Centers for Disease Control and Prevention. June 29, 2023. https://www.cdc.gov/violenceprevention/aces/index.html

5. Abramson A. How COVID-19 may increase domestic violence and child abuse. American Psychological Association. 2022. Accessed June 8, 2022. https://www.apa.org/topics/covid-19/domestic-violence-child-abuse

6. National child maltreatment statistics. American SPCC. 2023. https://americanspcc.org/child-maltreatment-statistics/#:~:text=4%20million%20child%20maltreatment%20referral,prevention%20%26%20post%2Dresponse%20services

7. Social determinants of health. US Department of Health and Humans Services. https://health.gov/healthypeople/priority-areas/social-determinants-health

8. Hunter AA, Flores G. Social determinants of health and child maltreatment: a systematic review. *Pediatr Res.* 2021;89(2):269-274. doi:10.1038/s41390-020-01175-x

9. Preventing child abuse and neglect. Centers for Disease Control and Prevention. 2021. Accessed June 8, 2022. https://www.cdc.gov/violenceprevention/childabuseandneglect/fastfact.html

10. Peterson C, Florence C, Klevens J. The economic burden of child maltreatment in the United States, 2015. *Child Abuse Negl.* 2018;86:178-183. doi:10.1007/s10560-020-00665-5

11. Lawson M, Piel MH, Simon M. Child maltreatment during the COVID-19 pandemic: consequences of parental job loss on psychological and physical abuse towards children. *Child Abuse Negl.* 2020;110:104709. doi:10.1016/j.chiabu.2020.104709

12. Pereda N, Díaz-Faes DA. Family violence against children in the wake of COVID-19 pandemic: a review of current perspectives and risk factors. *Child Adolesc Psychiatry Ment Health.* 2020;14(40). doi:10.1186/s13034-020-00347-1

13. Szarkowski A, Fogler J. Supporting students with disabilities in trauma-sensitive schools. Association for Supervision and Curriculum Development (ASCD). 2020. Accessed June 8, 2022. https://www.ascd.org/el/articles/supporting-students-with-disabilities-in-trauma-sensitive-schools

14. Risk and protective factors. Centers for Disease Control and Prevention. 2021. Accessed June 8, 2022. https://www.cdc.gov/violenceprevention/childabuseandneglect/riskprotectivefactors.html

15. Moving forward. Centers for Disease Control and Prevention. 2021. Accessed June 8, 2022. https://www.cdc.gov/violenceprevention/communicationresources/videos.html#childAbuseandNeglect

16. Mallett X, Schall U. The psychological and physiological sequel of child maltreatment: a forensic perspective. *Neurol Psychiatry Brain Res.* 2019;34:9-12. doi:10.1016/j.npbr.2019.08.003

17. Intimate partner violence and child abuse considerations during COVID-19. Substance Abuse and Mental Health Services Administration. https://www.samhsa.gov/sites/default/files/social-distancing-domestic-violence.pdf

18. How COVID-19 may increase domestic violence and child abuse. American Psychological Association. 2020. https://www.apa.org/topics/covid-19/domestic-violence-child-abuse

19. Trauma and violence. Substance Abuse and Mental Health Services Administration. 2022. Accessed June 8, 2022. https://www.samhsa.gov/trauma-violence

20. McEwan BS, Akil H. Revisiting the stress concept: implications for affective disorders. *J Neurosci.* 2020;40(1):12-21. doi:10.1523/JNEUROSCI.0733-19.2019

21. Smith KE, Pollak SD. Early life stress and development: potential mechanisms for adverse outcomes. *J Neurodev Disord.* 2020;12(34). doi:10.1186/s11689-020-09337-y

22. PACEs science 101 (FAQs) – positive and adverse childhood experiences. PACEsConnection. 2022. https://www.pacesconnection.com/blog/aces-101-faqs

23. Positive childhood experiences: how to reduce the impact of stress for children. American SPCC. 2023. https://americanspcc.org/positive-childhood-experience/

24. Protective factors to promote well-being and prevent child abuse and neglect. Child Welfare Information Gateway. 2020. Accessed June 8, 2022. https://www.childwelfare.gov/topics/preventing/promoting/protectfactors/

25. Mortazavi SS, Assari S, Alimohamadi A, Rafiee M, Shati M. Fear, loss, social isolation, and incomplete grief due to COVID-19: a recipe for a psychiatric pandemic. *Basic Clin Neurosci.* 2020;11(2):225-232. doi:10.32598/bcn.11.covid19.2549.1

26. Parrott DJ, Halmos MB, Stappenbeck CA, Moino K. Intimate partner aggression during the COVID-19 pandemic: associations with stress and heavy drinking. *Psychol Violence.* 2022;12(2):95-103. doi:10.1037/vio0000395

27. Piquero AR, Jennings WG, Jemison E, Kaukinen C, Knaul FM. Domestic violence during the COVID-19 pandemic - evidence from a systematic review and meta-analysis. *J Crim Justice.* 2021;74:101806. doi:10.1016/j.jcrimjus.2021.101806

28. Helping children cope after a traumatic event. Child Mind Institute. 2023. https://childmind.org/guide/helping-children-cope-after-a-traumatic-event/

29. Disaster technical assistance center supplemental research bulletin: behavioral health conditions in children and youth exposed to natural disasters. Substance Abuse and Mental Health Services Administration. 2018. https://www.samhsa.gov/sites/default/files/srb-childrenyouth-8-22-18.pdf

30. Warning signs and risk factors for emotional distress. Substance Abuse and Mental Health Services Administration. 2023. https://www.samhsa.gov/find-help/disaster-distress-helpline/warning-signs-risk-factors

31. Helping young children and parents transition back to school. Centers for Disease Control and Prevention. 2023. https://www.cdc.gov/childrensmentalhealth/features/COVID-19-helping-children-transition-back-to-school.html

32. 5 steps for brain-building serve and return. Harvard University: Center on the Developing Child. 2023. https://developingchild.harvard.edu/resources/5-steps-for-brain-building-serve-and-return/#:~:text=Child%2Dadult%20relationships%20that%20are,it%20takes%20two%20to%20play!

33. Trucco EM, Fava NM, Villar MG, Kumar M, Sutherland MT. Social isolation during the COVID-19 pandemic impacts the link between child abuse and adolescent internalizing problems. *J Youth Adolesc.* 2023;52(6):1313-1324. doi:10.1007/s10964-023-01775-w

34. Sprang G, Eslinger J, Whitt-Woosley A, et al. Child traumatic stress and COVID-19: the impact of the pandemic on a clinical sample of children in trauma

treatment. *J Child Adol Trauma.* 2023;16(3):659-670. doi:10.1007/s40653-023-00531-3

35. Moore DM. The impact of social isolation and COVID-19 pandemic mitigation on child welfare and domestic violence. CornerHouse. 2020. https://www.cornerhousemn.org/the-latest/the-impact-of-social-isolation-and-covid-19-pandemic-mitigation-on-child-welfare-and-domestic-violence

Chapter 5

SOCIAL DETERMINANTS OF HEALTH

Clariana Vitória Ramos de Oliveira, PhD, MSc, RN

OBJECTIVES

After reading this chapter, the reader will be able to:

1. *Understand the social determinants of health (SDHs) concepts.*

2. *Apply theories related to SDHs and child maltreatment to clinical practice.*

3. *Describe the relationship between child maltreatment and health.*

BACKGROUND AND SIGNIFICANCE

The environments to which individuals are exposed can influence lifelong developmental, physical, and mental health outcomes. SDHs, such as living and working conditions, interpersonal relationships between children, parents, and peers, family sociodemographics, learning environments, access to green spaces, neighborhood characteristics, cultural perspectives, violence exposure, and sociopolitical situations, affect people's lives on different levels, interact with one another, and represent a wide range of characteristics that are not of a biological foundation but rather are well established interactions between individuals' social and physical environments.

The initial stages of life, encompassing conception, pregnancy, and the post-natal phases, wield a substantial influence on the trajectories of health that extend across an individual's entire lifespan. The vulnerabilities experienced during these stages result from a complex interplay between development and social determinants. There are influences from the surrounding environment that shape the brain and refine executive functions, which produce a range of positive and negative stimuli that will continue throughout childhood, adolescence, and adulthood.

The extent to which these processes lead to healthy development depends upon the qualities of relationship, support, and nurturance in the social environments in which children live, learn, and grow. The potential for intervention to alleviate social inequities in health to improve the development outcomes of populations has led to researchers, governments, and policymakers progressively attempting to better understand the social conditions relating to child maltreatment.

Many children are exposed to social stressors that coexist at the individual, community, and societal levels, such as poverty, community violence, witnessing domestic violence, and maltreatment. Such adverse conditions are likely to contribute to undesirable child developmental trajectories and wellbeing. Additionally, the far-reaching effects of COVID-19 have led to a significant upsurge in reports of child maltreatment. The reality is that children exposed to one type of violence are often exposed to other types in the same developmental period or successively.[1,2]

The bioecological model of human development highlights how the multiple systems in which people live are interconnected and shape their development and how individual behaviors are affected by both individual and environmental characteristics.[3]

Identifying how contextual exposures can influence health and interact with family and individual-level characteristics as well as broader social systems is a crucial component of social epidemiological theories of disease distribution.[4] Strong relationships between social inequalities and child maltreatment serve as constant reminders of the necessity to understand how the settings in which we live, work, and socialize affect child health, development, and the relationship between children and caregivers.[4,5]

A THEORY OVERVIEW

BRONFENBRENNER

Urie Bronfenbrenner's bioecological model, often referred to as the ecological systems theory, provides a comprehensive framework for understanding child development.[3] This theory underscores the interplay of various ecological systems, each contributing to the child's development in unique ways. At the core of this model is the microsystem, which includes the immediate environments where a child is actively engaged. This encompasses family, school, peers, and other settings where children form essential social bonds. Beyond the microsystem is the exosystem, comprising environments indirectly impacting a child. This includes the community, neighborhood, and institutions such as health care systems or local policies, which can influence the resources and opportunities available to the child. In the mesosystem, a person's individual microsystems are not isolated entities but instead interact and impact each other. This interaction involves various microsystems within a child's life. For example, the relationship between a child's school and their family is part of the mesosystem. If a child is experiencing challenges at school, it may affect their interactions at home, and vice versa. The macrosystem extends to the broader societal and cultural contexts, encompassing political, social, economic, legal, and cultural factors. These elements establish the overarching framework within which the other systems operate. The chronosystem introduces the element of time, acknowledging that these systems change and evolve. How long a child is exposed to specific environments within these systems significantly impacts their development.

For practitioners, understanding the ecological systems allows them to make informed decisions when working with children and families. By considering the microsystem, practitioners can tailor interventions to the child's immediate environment, ensuring they are relevant and effective. This system-based perspective helps in creating strategies that align with the child's unique circumstances.

Policymakers can benefit from this model by recognizing the particular importance of the exosystem in shaping child development. By addressing factors in the exosystem, such as community resources, health care access, and social policies, policymakers can implement preventative strategies to support children and families. These measures can help reduce disparities and ensure that all children have equitable opportunities for growth and development. Policymakers can create changes in the macrosystem through changes in laws, influencing social norms, and cultural practices that positively impact children. For instance, changes in family leave policies, educational practices, and anti-discrimination laws can significantly influence children's wellbeing.

Practitioners and policymakers may consider forecasting how changes in the child's environment may affect their development and creating policies and interventions that adapt to evolving circumstances. This holistic perspective enables practitioners and policymakers to adopt more effective, holistic approaches to child wellbeing.

In essence, Bronfenbrenner's bioecological model helps practitioners and policymakers appreciate the multidimensional nature of child development. It encourages them to address not just individual behavior or isolated issues but to consider the complex interplay of systems that influence a child's growth and wellbeing. By doing so, they can create more effective, well rounded, and sustainable strategies for promoting positive child development.

BELSKY

Belsky's model[6,7] provides a comprehensive understanding of the determinants of parenting by highlighting the intricate interplay between parental developmental history, child characteristics, and social environments. This model introduces the concept of "contexts of maltreatment," recognizing various risk and protective factors within distinct domains related to the child, parent, family, and community.[6] This model can predict whether or not a child will experience maltreatment based on their age, health and behavior, parental childhood experiences and emotional stability, parent's mental health, patterns of family interaction, societal attitudes and practices regarding child rearing, and cultural beliefs that promote child maltreatment.

What is noteworthy is how Belsky's theory integrates seamlessly with Bronfenbrenner's ecological systems theory, expanding upon its four systems while excluding the chronosystem. Belsky's model incorporates the ontogenic system, which explores a parent's history of maltreatment, recognizing that a parent's abusive childhood environment might lead to replicating such an environment for their own child. The microsystem highlights the child's immediate family setting and the quality of their relationships within this context. The exosystem includes larger social structures exerting indirect influences on the family, encompassing factors like parental employment conditions, family poverty, parents' social networks, and social isolation.[6]

Moreover, Belsky's model underscores how the socio-condition of the family and the specific characteristics of the local neighborhood, such as violence, green spaces, and poverty, significantly contribute to the variation in child abuse rates within different neighborhoods. This integration of Belsky's model with Bronfenbrenner's ecological systems theory creates a holistic framework that illuminates the intricate dynamics between parent-child interactions, immediate family contexts, broader social structures, and community-specific variables in the context of child maltreatment.[7]

SDHs Associated with Child Maltreatment

Child maltreatment has been influenced by numerous distal determinants related to societal beliefs, political conditions, cultural aspects of the family, and wealth. Family poverty, for example, may impact the way parents interact with their children, as it increases the amount of stress experienced by the family and creates a hostile environment for the child.[8] Certainly, the concept of SDHs and their association with child maltreatment is a critical area of study. SDHs are external factors, beyond individual biology and genetics, that influence people's health and wellbeing.[9] These determinants encompass a wide range of social, economic, and environmental factors, and understanding their impact on child maltreatment is pivotal.[9] Research consistently shows that environmental risk factors can significantly influence child maltreatment.[5,7] These risk factors extend beyond the boundaries of the family system and reach into the broader societal context. The interaction between the family environment and these external risk factors is complex, and their cumulative impact can lead to a heightened risk of child maltreatment.[5,7]

Several key aspects are worth exploring in this context:

— **Poverty.** Lack of access to quality education and limited economic opportunities can place tremendous stress on families. Parents facing these challenges may experience heightened frustration, stress, and difficulty meeting the basic needs of their children, all of which can contribute to an increased risk of child maltreatment.

— **Community characteristics.** The neighborhood and community where a family resides play a significant role. Neighborhoods with high crime rates, a lack of social support networks, and limited access to essential services can all increase the likelihood of child maltreatment. Furthermore, neighborhoods with limited recreational opportunities or green spaces may reduce positive outlets for both parents and children.

— *Parental wellbeing.* The mental health and emotional stability of parents are key determinants of child maltreatment. High levels of parental stress, untreated mental health issues, or a history of maltreatment in the parent's own childhood can increase the risk.

— *Societal norms and attitudes.* Prevailing attitudes within a society regarding child rearing practices, discipline, and gender roles can also influence child maltreatment rates. In societies where violence as a form of discipline is more acceptable, or where rigid gender roles influence parenting responsibilities, child maltreatment may be more prevalent.

— *Social support.* The availability of social support networks, including family, friends, and community organizations, can act as a protective factor. Social support can reduce the risk of child maltreatment by providing parents with resources, advice, and assistance when needed.

These social determinants interact with one another, and the cumulative impact on families can be profound. Research that explores these relationships not only highlights the complexity of child maltreatment but also underscores the importance of comprehensive, multisystemic interventions. Understanding the role of SDHs in child maltreatment is crucial for policymakers and practitioners in developing effective strategies to mitigate the risk and provide support to vulnerable families. This chapter presents 3 dimensions that classify the SDHs, as illustrated in **Figure 5-1**.

***Figure 5-1.** A conceptual model for the illustration of social determinants and child maltreatment*

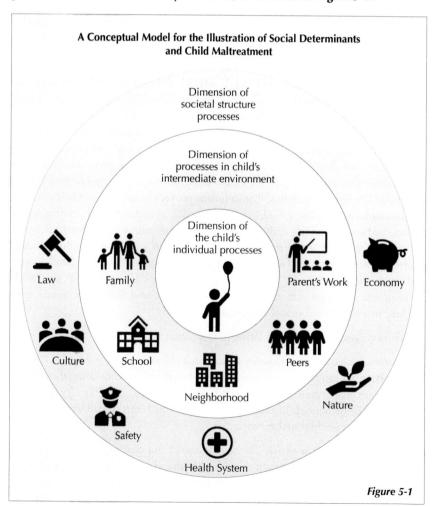

A Conceptual Model for the Illustration of Social Determinants and Child Maltreatment

Dimension of societal structure processes

Dimension of processes in child's intermediate environment

Dimension of the child's individual processes

Law · Family · Parent's Work · Economy · Culture · School · Neighborhood · Peers · Nature · Safety · Health System

Figure 5-1

The Dimension of Societal Structure Processes

The societal dimension is characterized by the broad aspects that influence and drive the structural forces of society.

Nature

Access to green spaces (eg, areas of grass, trees, or other vegetation, such as parks) is crucial in a child's development and behavioral health.[10] Green environments may positively affect wellbeing and emotional health[11,12] and mitigate stress in not only children, but also adults.[13] Caregivers exposed to green spaces are more likely to present psychological relaxation and stress alleviation, increased physical activity, and reduced exposure to air pollutants, noise, and excess heat.[14]

Stress reduction may support the parents' abilities to apply positive discipline when the child is misbehaving instead of physical or psychological punitive strategies. Additionally, neighborhoods that are safe, walkable, and have high-quality green spaces are associated with a greater frequency of behaviors that facilitate a positive social relationship between the child and caregiver.[15] Additionally, neighborhoods with high proportions of nature to yard space and less street traffic are associated with lower odds of young children experiencing emotional and social vulnerability,[16] such as maltreatment. However, green spaces must be accompanied by a safe place for the child to play and develop. In the United States, researchers found a correlation between the availability of green spaces in the neighborhood and children's vulnerability, which may be due to these spaces' lack of quality and supervision.[17]

Culture

Understanding the cultural aspects of child/caregiver relationships is crucial for comprehending child maltreatment perceptions. Cultural groups diverge in their interpretations of child maltreatment and children's misbehavior, potentially impacting the distinction between maltreatment and discipline.[18] Many cultures view children as inferior and prone to bad behavior, often leading to abusive punishments. Recognizing the influence of cultural backgrounds is vital for ensuring children's safety and wellbeing.

Cultural norms significantly shape parenting practices, with varying expectations regarding discipline and family roles. Some cultures emphasize strict discipline as a means of teaching respect, while others prioritize nurturing and emotional support. For instance, in some cultures, girls may be punished for not meeting family expectations related to chores and sibling care, while boys may be exposed to early sexual initiation.[19,20] These factors can signify maltreatment, potentially harming child development.

Respecting cultural diversity is essential to accommodating diverse parenting approaches, as long as the practices do not endanger children. Professionals working with families must be culturally sensitive, aiming for cultural competence. This involves understanding and appreciating cultural values and adapting services to be culturally sensitive. This approach fosters effective communication, collaboration, and child protection within the context of cultural backgrounds.

Ultimately, recognizing and respecting cultural and ethnic backgrounds is integral to child protection. Acknowledging cultural nuances allows providers and advocates to engage with families in a sensitive manner, facilitating dialogue while safeguarding children's wellbeing. Cultural competence, combined with advocating for children's rights, contributes to nurturing children's health, respecting cultural diversity, and promoting their overall wellbeing.

Poverty

Community poverty, characterized by low family income, is a significant risk factor for increasing family stress, housing vulnerability, and exposure to child violence.[21]

The mechanisms by which poverty is associated with child maltreatment remain unclear, although some evidence suggests that deprivation can influence negative parental behaviors toward children.[22,23] A lack of resources may also interfere with the economic decision for adequate child care, thereby resulting in an increased chance of child maltreatment.[24]

It has also been suggested that the psychological symptoms experienced by parents who are suffering from financial stress decrease levels of sensitive and supportive parenting behaviors.[22] Overall, the literature suggests that poverty has significant associations with child maltreatment.[24-28] Drake & Jonson-Reid,[29] for example, found that children in poverty are 3 times more likely to be maltreated than children in higher-income households.

Consequently, it becomes evident that effective interventions aimed at preventing child maltreatment should adopt a holistic approach. Identifying at-risk families is just the initial step, and it is equally crucial to address the underlying economic strains and challenges they face. This dual-pronged strategy, which combines support for economic stability with comprehensive parenting education and assistance, holds significant promise in breaking the cycle of maltreatment and promoting child wellbeing across all socioeconomic strata.

Addressing economic hardship through targeted assistance programs, such as financial counseling, affordable housing initiatives, or access to vocational training, can have far-reaching effects. By mitigating the financial stressors experienced by families, these interventions not only improve their economic wellbeing but also alleviate a critical risk factor for child maltreatment.

By integrating economic support with parenting education, communities can foster a more comprehensive approach to child wellbeing. This approach not only benefits individual families but also contributes to the overall social fabric, ultimately reducing the prevalence of child maltreatment and promoting healthier and more supportive environments for children to thrive. Such an approach takes a substantial step towards safeguarding the rights and wellbeing of every child, regardless of their socioeconomic background.

THE DIMENSION OF PROCESSES IN THE CHILD'S INTERMEDIATE ENVIRONMENT

The intermediate dimension is characterized by where the child lives, which thereby affects the family's life as a whole and whether the child may be directly exposed to violence or not.

NEIGHBORHOOD

The community where families are situated is impacted by a variety of risk and protective factors for maltreatment. The interactions between children and caregivers are based not only on their own experiences but also on the settings and social and structural forces in which they are situated.[5] The surrounding contexts of the family, including community centers, schools, churches, health centers, and neighbors, are necessary for establishing a support network and creating strong communities that prevent child maltreatment.[30] Certain neighborhood characteristics, such as high levels of violence, low adult-to-child ratios, concentrated disadvantage, and high population density, have been linked to increased instances of child maltreatment. Conversely, protective factors, such as interconnected members, intergenerational closure (ie, a social network in which a child's parent knows the parents of the child's friends), and high social networks, have been associated with lower proportions of abuse and neglect.[31]

This complex dynamic between the factors contributing to child maltreatment extends further to include the interplay of collective efficacy, social disorder, and their impacts on individual and community wellbeing. Collective efficacy, a concept encapsulating a group's shared belief in their collective capabilities to succeed in various tasks, plays a pivotal role in the dynamics of child maltreatment. In communities where collective efficacy is strong, individuals are more likely to come together to address common issues, including child safety, thereby acting as a protective factor against maltreatment. In addition, communities grappling with greater levels of violence and social disorder often face challenges in nurturing collective efficacy. High rates of community violence, limited social capital, extensive policing activity, housing instability (as indicated by rent burden), a high percentage of persons with disabilities, and concentrated neighborhood disadvantage have been identified as risk factors for child maltreatment.[32-34] These risk factors paint a complex picture of the social processes at play within communities. The influence of these social processes on child maltreatment is both direct and indirect.[24,31] For example, communities marred by violence and disorder can create environments of heightened stress, impacting parenting behaviors. Parents living in such neighborhoods may face increased parenting stress and diminished internal control, potentially increasing the risk of child maltreatment. These challenges not only affect the family dynamics but also erode the community's ability to mobilize collective efficacy in support of child wellbeing.

Understanding the intricate relationships between collective efficacy, social disorder, individual characteristics, and community dynamics is vital for designing effective interventions. These interventions should aim to not only strengthen the protective factors within communities but also address the underlying challenges contributing to social disorder and violence. By fostering collective efficacy, promoting social capital, and alleviating neighborhood disadvantage, professionals can work towards creating environments where child maltreatment is less likely to occur. In this way, they not only improve individual and community wellbeing, but also uphold the fundamental rights and safety of children.

PARENT EMPLOYMENT CONDITION

The parent's employment conditions are highly interrelated with child maltreatment but are still conceptually and empirically associated with socioeconomic characteristics.[35] For example, parental education, occupation, unemployment (ie, no remunerative work), housing, and poverty are all considered as potentially modifiable factors that contribute to economic disadvantage and are linked to parents' behavior.[35] Little research has been conducted on the impact of parental employment, employment benefits (eg, parental leave, child care assistance, sick days), and employment conditions (eg, skilled trades versus manual labor jobs) on children. The importance of parent employment was evident in a study that observed parents' work situations during COVID-19 and found that it was a significant risk factor for child maltreatment.[36] The researcher found that parents experiencing depression and job loss were more likely to psychologically and physically maltreat their children.[36] Furthermore, a different study showed that in families with a low socioeconomic status or parental unemployment, physical abuse is 3 times higher and the risk of neglect is 7 times higher.[37]

PARENTAL MENTAL ILLNESS

Researchers found an increased chance of child maltreatment when the mother has a mental illness, even once the study's sociodemographic characteristics have been controlled for.[25,38] Parental mental illness affects parents' capacity to adequately protect their children due to the difficulties they experience in organizing their lives, controlling their emotions, attending to their children's physical needs, and being emotionally responsive.[39] Another mental health trait indicative of potential maltreatment is the maternal acknowledgment of early-life maltreatment in a child, such as incidents involving shaking.[40]

Domestic Violence

Children's exposure to domestic violence, whether directly witnessed or overheard, is harmful and may lead to post-traumatic stress disorder and other severe emotional and behavioral difficulties.[41] Further, intimate partner violence and child abuse often co-occur, and children will likely experience an increased risk of maltreatment when isolated at home.[42] It is estimated that in 1/2 of the cases of intimate partner violence, one or both caregivers are aggressive toward the child.[43] Family violence is also associated with a range of factors, including economic stress, disaster-related instability, increased exposure to exploitative relationships, and reduced options for support.[44]

The Dimension of the Child's Individual Processes

Child Characteristics

At the closest level of the social determinants of maltreatment are the unique characteristics of the child. While some may not categorize child characteristics as conventional social determinants, many researchers, including those cited in this context, do consider them integral to understanding the individual risk factors associated with child maltreatment. These factors are important to recognize and address, as they can significantly impact a child's wellbeing and safety.

One important child-level determinant linked to child maltreatment is a child's health status. Studies have shown that children with low birth weights or those born with congenital diseases are at increased risk of maltreatment.[45] These factors not only contribute to poor health and developmental outcomes but can also make these children more vulnerable to maltreatment. Such children may require additional care and support, which can exacerbate stress levels within families, potentially leading to maltreatment.

Another determinant is the child's age and developmental stage.[9] A child's age and developmental stage are vital considerations. Infants and very young children may be more vulnerable due to their dependency on caregivers, while older children may face unique challenges related to schooling, peer relationships, and autonomy. Understanding age-related risks and protective factors is essential.

The child's temperament and behavior,[46] including traits like adaptability and activity level, can influence parenting practices. Children with difficult temperaments may experience increased parenting stress, potentially leading to maltreatment. Recognizing and addressing these differences is crucial.

Children with special needs represent another group at higher risk for maltreatment.[47,48] Their unique requirements, whether due to physical, cognitive, or emotional challenges, can strain a caregiver's coping abilities, especially if adequate support services are lacking. Children with special educational needs, such as learning disabilities, attention-deficit/hyperactivity disorder, or autism spectrum disorder, may require additional support in school and at home. Their unique challenges can increase stress within families. Adequate educational services and family support are essential. This added burden can contribute to heightened parenting stress and, in some cases, maltreatment.[47]

Children who have had contact with child welfare agencies are also identified as being at risk of maltreatment.[49] This group includes children who have been involved in the child protection system due to concerns for their safety and wellbeing. Previous interactions with child welfare agencies may suggest ongoing challenges within the family, which can contribute to maltreatment risks. Likewise, children who have experienced trauma, such as abuse, neglect, or witnessing violence, are at increased risk of maltreatment. Recognizing past trauma and providing trauma-informed care can help break the cycle of maltreatment.

A child's social network, including relationships with peers and adults outside of the family, can be protective factors. Building healthy social connections for children can reduce their risk of maltreatment, and resilience factors such as coping skills and a strong self-concept can act as protective mechanisms for children. Promoting resilience through supportive environments and interventions can enhance a child's ability to withstand adversity.

Addressing these child-level determinants requires a holistic and individualized approach. It involves providing tailored support and interventions based on the child's specific needs, developmental stage, and family context. By recognizing and addressing these factors, practitioners, policymakers, and advocates can work towards creating safer environments for children and preventing child maltreatment effectively.

Conclusion

Child maltreatment is a complex issue influenced by different family and societal dynamics, affecting the child's intermediate and proximal environment. In clinical settings, it is critical that the clinician consider the chain of SDHs and investigate the child's history with a holistic lens when evaluating for the risk of maltreatment. In other settings, policymakers and related professionals must recognize the inherent complexity of child maltreatment and use this recognition to direct their attention to social context factors, which are manifested in the nurturing and care provided to a child. Such attention should lead professionals to enact and continue developing effective and family-centered interventions.

Key Points

1. Child maltreatment is a multifaceted issue influenced by different family and societal dynamics that affect the child's intermediate and proximal environment.

2. There are several theories related to the social determinants of child development and maltreatment, such as Bronfenbrenner's and Belsky's, that outline the associated risk and protective factors.

3. Understanding the influence of social determinants on child maltreatment is crucial to providing quality care and support to survivors.

References

1. Cuartas J, Grogan-Kaylor A, Ma J, Castillo B. Civil conflict, domestic violence, and poverty as predictors of corporal punishment in Colombia. *Child Abuse Negl*. 2019;90:108-119. doi:10.1016/j.chiabu.2019.02.003

2. Hamby S, Finkelhor D, Turner H, Ormrod R. The overlap of witnessing partner violence with child maltreatment and other victimizations in a nationally representative survey of youth. *Child Abuse Negl*. 2010;34(10):734-741. doi:10.1016/j.chiabu.2010.03.001

3. Bronfenbrenner U, Morris P. The bioecological model of human development. In: Damon W, Lerner RM, eds. *Handbook of Child Psychology*. 6th ed. John Wiley & Sons, Inc; 2007.

4. Arcaya MC, Tucker-Seeley RD, Kim R, Schnake-Mahl A, So M, Subramanian SV. Research on neighborhood effects on health in the United States: a systematic review of study characteristics. *Soc Sci Med*. 2016;168:16-29. doi:10.1016/j.socscimed.2016.08.047

5. Cuartas J. Neighborhood crime undermines parenting: violence in the vicinity of households as a predictor of aggressive discipline. *Child Abuse Negl*. 2018;76:388-399. doi:10.1016/j.chiabu.2017.12.006

6. Bronfenbrenner U. *The Ecology of Human Development: Experiments by Nature and Design*. Harvard University Press; 1979.

7. Belsky J. Etiology of child maltreatment: a developmental-ecological analysis. *Psychol Bull.* 1993;114(3):413-434. doi:10.1037/0033-2909.114.3.413

8. Ho LLK, Li WHC, Cheung AT, Luo Y, Xia W, Chung JOK. Impact of poverty on parent-child relationships, parental stress, and parenting practices. *Front Public Health.* 2022;10:849408. doi:10.3389/fpubh.2022.849408

9. Font SA, Berger LM. Child maltreatment and children's developmental trajectories in early to middle childhood. *Child Dev.* 2015;86(2):536-556. doi:10.1111/cdev.12322

10. Jung H, Herrenkohl TI, Lee JO, Hemphill SA, Heerde JA, Skinner ML. Gendered pathways from child abuse to adult crime through internalizing and externalizing behaviors in childhood and adolescence. *J Interpers Violence.* 2017;32(18):2724-2750. doi:10.1177/0886260515596146

11. Markevych I, Tiesler CM, Fuertes E, et al. Access to urban green spaces and behavioural problems in children: results from the GINIplus and LISAplus studies [published correction appears in Environ Int. 2015 Sep;82:115]. *Environ Int.* 2014;71:29-35. doi:10.1016/j.envint.2014.06.002

12. Richardson EA, Pearce J, Mitchell R, Kingham S. Role of physical activity in the relationship between urban green space and health. *Public Health.* 2013;127(4):318-324. doi:10.1016/j.puhe.2013.01.004

13. Bowler DE, Buyung-Ali LM, Knight TM, Pullin AS. A systematic review of evidence for the added benefits to health of exposure to natural environments. *BMC Public Health.* 2010;10:456. doi:10.1186/1471-2458-10-456

14. Fan Y, Das KV, Chen Q. Neighborhood green, social support, physical activity, and stress: assessing the cumulative impact. *Health Place.* 2011;17(6):1202-1211. doi:10.1016/j.healthplace.2011.08.008

15. Urban green spaces and health: a review of evidence. World Health Organization, Regional Office for Europe. 2016. https://www.who.int/europe/publications/i/item/WHO-EURO-2016-3352-43111-60341

16. Christian H, Zubrick SR, Foster S, et al. The influence of the neighborhood physical environment on early child health and development: a review and call for research. *Health Place.* 2015;33:25-36. doi:10.1016/j.healthplace.2015.01.005

17. Christian H, Ball SJ, Zubrick SR, et al. Relationship between the neighbourhood built environment and early child development. *Health Place.* 2017;48:90-101. doi:10.1016/j.healthplace.2017.08.010

18. Bell MF, Turrell G, Beesley B, et al. Children's neighbourhood physical environment and early development: an individual child level linked data study. *J Epidemiol Community Health.* 2020;74(4):321-329. doi:10.1136/jech-2019-212686

19. Ninsiima AB, Leye E, Michielsen K, Kemigisha E, Nyakato VN, Coene G. "Girls Have More Challenges; They Need to Be Locked Up": a qualitative study of gender norms and the sexuality of young adolescents in Uganda. *Int J Environ Res Public Health.* 2018;15(2):193. doi:10.3390/ijerph15020193

20. Weber AM, Cislaghi B, Meausoone V, et al. Gender norms and health: insights from global survey data. *Lancet.* 2019;393(10189):2455-2468. doi:10.1016/S0140-6736(19)30765-2

21. Cho M. A prospective, longitudinal cohort study: the impact of child maltreatment on delinquency among South Korean youth in middle and high school. *Child Abuse Negl.* 2019;88:235-245. doi:10.1016/j.chiabu.2018.11.021

22. Barboza G, Appel JG. Child maltreatment data in the state of New Mexico across space and time. *Data Brief.* 2020;31:105759. doi:10.1016/j.dib.2020.105759

23. Newland RP, Crnic KA, Cox MJ, Mills-Koonce WR; Family Life Project Key Investigators. The family model stress and maternal psychological symptoms: mediated pathways from economic hardship to parenting. *J Fam Psychol.* 2013; 27(1):96-105. doi:10.1037/a0031112

24. Schenck-Fontaine A, Gassman-Pines A. Income inequality and child maltreatment risk during economic recession. *Children Youth Serv Rev.* 2020;112(47): 104926. doi:10.1016/j.childyouth.2020.104926

25. Maguire-Jack K, Font SA. Community and individual risk factors for physical child abuse and child neglect: variations by poverty status. *Child Maltreat.* 2017;22(3):215-226. doi:10.1177/1077559517711806

26. Baldwin H, Biehal N, Allgar V, Cusworth L, Pickett K. Antenatal risk factors for child maltreatment: linkage of data from a birth cohort study to child welfare records. *Child Abuse Negl.* 2020;107:104605. doi:10.1016/j.chiabu.2020.104605

27. Biehal N, Cusworth L, Hooper J, Whincup H, Shapira M. Pathways to permanence for children who become looked after in Scotland. University of Stirling. 2019. https://www.stir.ac.uk/research/public-policy-hub/policy-briefings/

28. Bywaters P, Brady G, Sparks T, Bos E. Child welfare inequalities: new evidence, further questions. *Child Fam Soc Work.* 2014;21:369-380. doi:10.1111/cfs.12154

29. Drake B, Jonson-Reid M. Poverty and child maltreatment. In: Korbin J, Krugman RD, eds. *Handbook of Child Maltreatment.* Springer; 2013.

30. Lepistö S, Ellonen N, Helminen M, Paavilainen E. The family health, functioning, social support and child maltreatment risk of families expecting a baby. *J Clin Nurs.* 2017;26(15-16):2439-2451. doi:10.1111/jocn.13602

31. van Dijken MW, Stams GJJM, Winter M. Can community-based interventions prevent child maltreatment? *Child Youth Serv Rev.* 2016;61:149-158. doi:10.1016/j.childyouth.2015.12.007

32. Molnar BE, Goerge RM, Gilsanz P, et al. Neighborhood-level social processes and substantiated cases of child maltreatment. *Child Abuse Negl.* 2016;51:41-53. doi:10.1016/j.chiabu.2015.11.007

33. Marco M, Maguire-Jack K, Gracia E, López-Quílez A. Disadvantaged neighborhoods and the spatial overlap of substantiated and unsubstantiated child maltreatment referrals. *Child Abuse Negl.* 2020;104:104477. doi:10.1016/j.chiabu.2020.104477

34. Barboza-Salerno GE. Variability and stability in child maltreatment risk across time and space and its association with neighborhood social and housing vulnerability in New Mexico: a bayesian space-time model. *Child Abuse Negl.* 2020;104:104472. doi:10.1016/j.chiabu.2020.104472

35. Gracia E, López-Quílez A, Marco M, Lila M. Mapping child maltreatment risk: a 12-year spatio-temporal analysis of neighborhood influences. *Int J Health Geogr.* 2017;16(1):38. doi:10.1186/s12942-017-0111-y

36. Doidge JC, Higgins DJ, Delfabbro P, et al. Economic predictors of child maltreatment in an Australian population-based birth cohort. *Child Youth Serv Rev.* 2017;72:14-25. doi:10.1016/j.childyouth.2016.10.012

37. Lawson M, Piel MH, Simon M. Child maltreatment during the COVID-19 pandemic: consequences of parental job loss on psychological and physical abuse

towards children. *Child Abuse Negl.* 2020;110(2):104709. doi:10.1016/j.chia-bu.2020.104709

38. Sedlak AJ, Mettenburg J, Basena M, et al. *Fourth National Incidence Study of Child Abuse and Neglect (NIS-4): Report to Congress, Executive Summary.* US Department of Health and Human Services, Administration for Children and Families; 2010.

39. White OG, Hindley N, Jones DP. Risk factors for child maltreatment recurrence: an updated systematic review. *Med Sci Law.* 2015;55(4):259-277. doi:10.1177/0025802414543855

40. Cleaver H, Unell I, Aldgate A. *Child Abuse: Parental Mental Illness, Learning Disability, Substance Misuse and Domestic Violence.* TSO; 2011.

41. Sakakihara A, Masumoto T, Kurozawa Y. The association between maternal shaking behavior and inappropriate infant parenting: the Japan environment and children's study. *Front Public Health.* 2022;10:848321. doi:10.3389/fpubh.2022.848321

42. Ravi KE, Casolaro TE. Children's exposure to intimate partner violence: a qualitative interpretive meta-synthesis. *Child Adolesc Soc Work J.* 2018;35:283-295. doi:10.1007/s10560-017-0525-1

43. Hamby S, Finkelhor D, Turner H, Ormrod R. The overlap of witnessing partner violence with child maltreatment and other victimizations in a nationally representative survey of youth. *Child Abuse Negl.* 2010;34:734-741. doi:10.1016/j.chiabu.2010.03.001

44. Jouriles EN, Rosenfield D, McDonald R, Vu NL, Rancher C, Mueller V. Children exposed to intimate partner violence: conduct problems, interventions, and partner contact with the child. *J Clin Child Adolesc Psychol.* 2018;47(3):397-409. doi:10.1080/15374416.2016.1163706

45. Peterman A, Potts A, O'Donnell M, et al. *Pandemics and Violence Against Women and Children. CGD Working Paper 528.* Center for Global Development; 2020. https://www.cgdev.org/publication/pandemics-and-violence-against-women-and-children

46. Pekdoğan S, Kanak M. Child temperament as a predictor of parents' potential for emotional abuse. *J Nerv Ment Dis.* 2022;210(5):330–334. doi:10.1097/NMD.0000000000001449

47. Kawaguchi H, Fujiwara T, Okamoto Y, et al. Perinatal determinants of child maltreatment in Japan. *Front Pediatr.* 2020;8:143-143. doi:10.3389/fped.2020.00143

48. Bartholet E, Wulczyn F, Barth RP, Lederman C. *Race and Child Welfare.* Chapin Hall at the University of Chicago; 2011.

49. Maltby LE, Callahan KL, Friedlander S, Shetgiri R. Infant temperament and behavioral problems: analysis of high-risk infants in child welfare. *J Public Child Welf.* 2019;13(5):512-528. doi:10.1080/15548732.2018.1536626

BIOGRAPHICAL TIMELINES

Beth I. Barol, PhD, LSW, BCB, NADD-CC
Sarah H. Buffie, MSW, LSW

OBJECTIVES

After reading this chapter, the reader will be able to:

1. *Understand the implications of planning interventions without sufficient exploration of biographical root causes of "challenging behaviors."*

2. *Describe the importance of biographical timelines as a framework to provide holistic, compassionate supports.*

3. *Recognize the impact of a caregiver, understanding their roles from the perspective of a social therapist.*

BACKGROUND AND SIGNIFICANCE

Children are often labeled, blamed, punished, and disregarded due to their overt behaviors. Punitive and pathologizing responses by caregivers and teachers only serve to exacerbate the problems. When making support plans based on a crisis, the larger context of the child's history may be missed. When someone is understood in the context of their life experiences, providers are able to build compassionate supports that are relevant to the person as a whole, instead of minimizing them to the sum of their "challenging behaviors."

Over the past 20 years, there have been many advances in our collective knowledge about the brain, the brain/body continuum, trauma and its treatment, physical and mental health diagnosis, new medications, genetics, genetic testing, and environmental factors as they relate to health and disability, among many others. This expansion of knowledge has had a direct impact on the treatment options available for those who access mental health services. Today, talking therapies are one modality used to help people heal; however, we now have a fuller appreciation of somatic therapies,[1] holistic health approaches, neurofeedback, and neuro entrainment[2] to promote certain frequencies in the brain.[3] The possibilities expand on a continuous basis with promising potentials to help people heal and recover from head injuries, traumas, neurological challenges, and mental illness.[4-7]

As exciting as these new discoveries and innovations are, clinicians have observed in their practice that there remains a wide gap between what is known or knowable and what is practiced or available to most of the population. The gap between knowledge and practice is wider still for children and adults who have intellectual and cognitive differences (ID) or who are members of underserved and marginalized populations and whose cultural and survival strategies may emerge as challenging behavioral patterns. There are relatively few clinicians and practitioners who are both skilled in the aforementioned advancements and are willing and able to offer their skills to children with challenging behavioral expressions. Many clinicians have said that the diagnosis of ID, for example, overshadows any other assessment of root causes for the observed challenging behavior. However, when professionals broaden their assessment beyond the context of ID and observable challenging behaviors, they can better invest time, resources, and compassion in noticing and addressing the root issues. These issues include the wide array of mental illness, trauma, and neurological differences, and the challenges of mentoring them to apply promising practices available to the neurotypical population to address the child's specific issues.

Focusing on the role of families and other direct supporters is one of the key means to ensure that many of the advances in knowledge and practice will become available to all children who experience maltreatment. The social therapist is the direct support person who, with training, mentoring, and support, implements promising practices, advocates for necessary services, and plays a vital role in the care team. However, the biographical timeline approach is what truly informs the transformation of a team's view of a person and generates a rich assessment of the wounds, issues, and missed opportunities that have contributed to the child's current struggles and challenging behaviors.

The Social Therapist

Anthroposophist Karl Koenig coined the term "social therapy" through the curative education focus of the international Camphill Movement.[5] While many who are considered social therapists are formally trained and licensed mental health professionals, it is not an official job title. As such, a social therapist can be a family member, direct care professional, friend, teacher, nurse, case worker, supports coordinator, or any other person who comes in regular contact with the individual and has the skills and training to intentionally plan for interactions, environments, and activities that promote the wellbeing, healing, and empowerment of those they are supporting.

With the exception of the person they are supporting, the social therapists are the most crucial members of the team. They are the ones who deeply know the person and are attuned to their rhythms, needs, joys, health, and the relevant details in their daily lives. Social therapists are the people who help the person experience warmth and are able to offer a positive mirror of themselves as they offer opportunities for the person they support to feel known, to feel emotionally seen and heard, to explore their environment safely, to develop new skills, and to grow when they are ready. They are skilled at timing, knowing when to invite opportunities for further growth—such as learning new skills and practicing mastered skills—and pause in the moment and offer support to help the person relax and unwind. They know when their immediate presence is necessary and when space and time to oneself is the preferable option.

Social therapists have an opportunity to give vital information to the rest of the therapy team to use when designing clinical and additional therapeutic supports. They help assure that the clinicians and other professionals have opportunity to apply their valuable skills in a person-centered manner, and they are the key to implementing a person-directed holistic support model, including attention to calming practices, exercise, and healthy nutrition. These are the people in one's daily life who are trustworthy, dependable, respectful, present, and compassionate. Through their relationships, social therapists help to provide an environment where a person is able to flourish and any additional therapeutic intervention that has a chance to make a meaningful impact.

All too often, direct supporters are not thought of as social therapists or as those who have the potential to be social therapists. They are seen as "babysitters," physical care providers, safety monitors, and behavior plan enforcers. While there are many agencies, facilities, and providers of services that do in fact focus on developing the social therapist, sadly, this vital component is often overlooked. Staff training is focused more on meeting regulations and safety procedures than on inspiration, knowledge enhancement, creative approaches to everyday situations, role modeling, and processing the day or week with an experienced mentor.

Direct supporters are often assigned to work with a person without knowing anything about the person except their challenging behaviors and the behavior plan designed to manage these behaviors. When this happens without training or ongoing mentoring and support, the direct supporters are often left to conceptualize their role as being responsible for containing or extinguishing the challenging behaviors without being afforded the opportunity to know the full context for these behaviors, their root causes, and even their purpose. As a result, direct service providers face children with challenging behaviors on a regular basis often without feeling that they have the skills or resources to feel safe and to make a positive difference. This can be very stressful, frustrating and intimidating for the support person, leading to burnout for friends and family members and frequent turnover of support staff. Their image of the person they are assigned to support often becomes reduced to disparaging labels such as "manipulative," "troublemaker," or "defiant," and perpetuates the myth that this person is different from anyone they can understand or relate to.

When demonizing and distancing occurs, there are several tools and processes that can be employed to help transform the relationship between the person being supported and their caregiver. One such framework is the "biographical timeline," a process that helps transform the caregivers into a social therapist working on the behalf of the person.

THE BIOGRAPHICAL TIMELINE

The biographical timeline is a tool used to achieve a deeper and more meaningful understanding of a patient in order to transform relationships and intervention approaches. It is a tool that works best when the entire team is present to examine the information gleaned from records, interviews, and first-hand knowledge about the person. Events and personal experiences that were previously stored in compartmentalized reports and files, often thought of as insignificant in other contexts, are grouped and examined according to their occurrence along a linear life-timeline (**Figure 6-1**).[8]

The facilitator will bring the team together and guide the group process as they glean information from the participating team members. Members should attempt to identify wounds (eg, painful emotional, relational, and physical experiences), issues (eg, traumatic or toxic stress, feeling unloved or unlovable, as well as being subjected to systemic barriers such as marginalization, labeling, bias, and overshadowing diagnosis as well as a lack of resources and problematic funding allocation choices), and missed opportunities in the person's life. Together they explore the meaning of these experiences and how they shape the person's worldview, sense of self, and their capacity for safe behavioral expression. This provides the members of the team with an opportunity to teach each other about trauma, neurological differences, and mental illness as well as healing modalities and daily practices as they relate to the subject of the biographical timeline. By filling in the knowledge gap, the social therapists and other team members are better prepared to creatively come up with daily life supports and make specific treatment recommendations. The 3 case studies at the end of the chapter demonstrate the increased potential of social therapists when they have the opportunity to build compassion in conjunction with training on elements specific to the person's biography and issues.

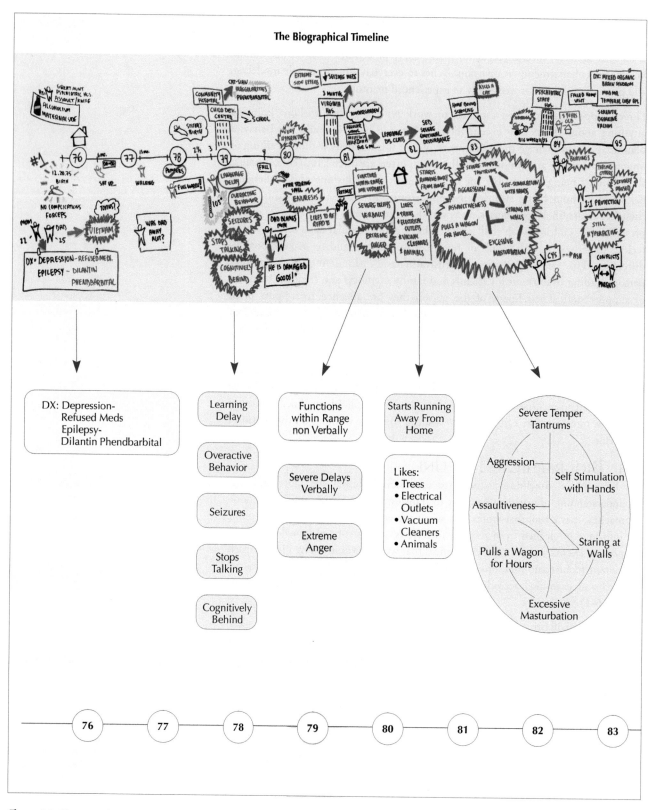

Figure 6-1. *The Biographical Timeline*

Follow-Up Steps

Following the biographical timeline session, best practice includes taking a 1/2 or full day where direct service workers and caregivers are supported in imagining themselves as social therapists. The team builds upon the compassion that results from the understanding of a person with a biographical timeline study. Facilitators guide the

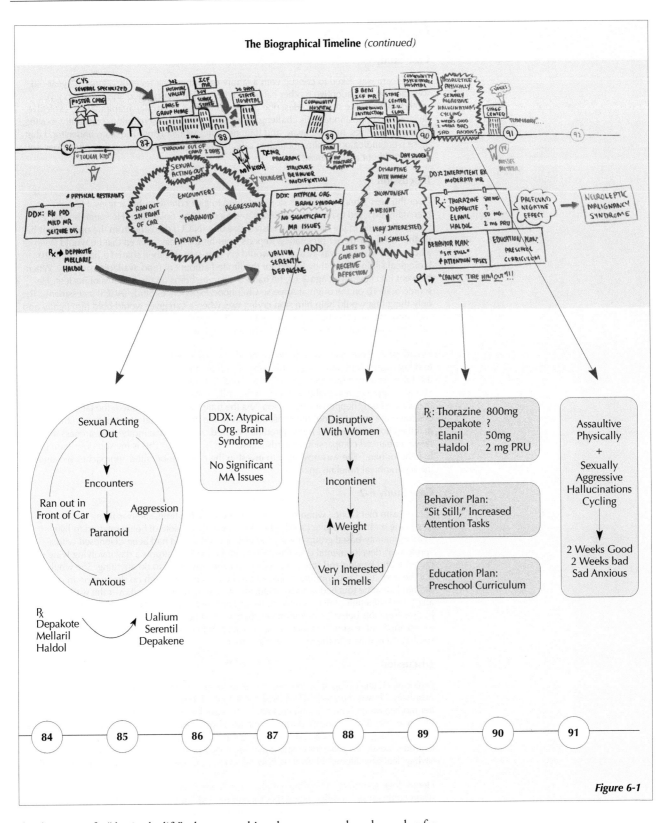

The Biographical Timeline *(continued)*

Figure 6-1

development of a "day in the life" where everything the supporters have learned so far is combined to build a sample day for the person, detailing the environment, home and community life, and design meaningful and purposeful action steps to build a life of love, belonging, safety, and mutually enhancing relationships, through the implementation of a 24-hour plan for a day.

CASE STUDIES

Case Study 6-1

A care team was asked to consult with a family regarding their recently adopted 3-year-old son, Jackson. The adoptive mother came into the session exasperated and "ready to give custody back to the state." To describe Jackson, she used words like manipulative, explosive, defiant, and oppositional. His challenging behaviors included screaming, constantly moving, hitting his siblings, running away, and flipping tables while raging. The team understood that these were indicators of him not feeling safe, but telling this to the caregivers often does not register without a full context.

Discussion

Over the next 2 hours, Jackson's story unfolded to give context to his actions. He was prenatally exposed to domestic violence and alcohol and opiate use. He spent the first 2 weeks of his life in the neonatal intensive care unit (NICU) detoxing from the opiates that his mother used during her pregnancy. Reports from his early days shared that he would sleep all day, and when he was awake, he would cry non-stop. He then shared a home with 20 biological siblings, and they fought for the limited amount of food available each day. When he went into custody at age 2 1/2, he had 78 cigarette burns on the bottoms of his feet. He scored a 10/10 on the original Adverse Childhood Experiences Study (ACES) assessment.[9] The only thing that would help him stop crying was when a caregiver would hold him tightly and rock him. The team realized that not only did these actions help in his infancy, but they were still something that he needed to feel safe and calm today at the age of 3.

His adoptive mom was ready to move ahead towards adoption, and her social services worker told her, "Just adopt him, change his name. He'll be fine. He won't remember a thing." Since this false assurance was given by a "professional," the adopting mother believed that myth. She was surprised and highly reactive to the child's ensuing challenging behaviors, claiming that they would "happen for no reason." As the timeline story continued, the facilitator educated the parents about the consequences to the brain, mental constructs, and the body that the abuse and neglect he endured had caused. The adoptive mother's awareness and newly enhanced compassion towards Jackson led her to say, "This is my son now, I am going to fight for him." She was now able to invest in the daily life-oriented approaches woven into the biographical timeline analysis.

Case Study 6-2

A care team met Donna when she was 7 years old. At the time, she was living on a cot in a living room in a respite care house and was in the middle of being referred to live in a community-based group home. She was nonverbal and had been diagnosed with a "profound" developmental disability. She would have 30 tantrums a day involving lying on the floor and kicking and screaming whenever she was asked to do anything. She would run out the door and keep running as fast and as far as she could with no destination in mind. She did not like to be touched or to eat food; she would color or draw all over the walls, rip things apart, and sometimes fall down the stairs and not even cry. She had multiple self-inflicted bruises from this behavior. Additionally, there were times where she would cry in the corner for no apparent reason. Previous caregivers labeled her as manipulative, noncompliant, spoiled, "a real pain in the neck," and a burden.

Discussion

Exploring Donna's biography led her care team to the root of her challenging behavioral expression. It was reported that while she was in her biological home and still in the crib, her mother would burn her with cigarettes and leave her alone for hours. Donna also had a history of grand mal seizures, during which her abusive mother likely left her unattended rather than providing adequate care. As the picture started to become clearer, the team noticed her tantrums looked a lot like these grand mal seizures. Donna's "tantrums" became her way of saying "leave me alone," illustrating how behavioral expression is a means of communication.

Her biological mother, struggling with her own mental health issues, eventually left the home when Donna was a toddler. Her father then remarried, and the new mother only knew Donna as an annoying child with tantrums. Wanting children of her own, she gave Donna's father an ultimatum, which led him to place his daughter in the foster care system.

Anxiety is a built-in defense mechanism that ensures human survival, but the dynamic between caregiver and child should teach children about trust, predictability, and the power of another's voice to respond and soothe. These patterned, repetitive experiences reduce the power of anxiety to its rightful small, but protective, function in the child's internal dynamic.[10]

By looking at a life from birth onward to understand someone's biography, providers and caregivers are able to pause and analyze the child's lived experience to better understand their divergent behaviors. The team should question the psychological impact of the following questions: What happens when someone is overcome by pain? What happens when someone has trouble breathing? How does that affect someone's faith in their own body? What is the meaning-making that begins to weave throughout the body's memories with experiences like these? What happens when someone cannot trust their caregiver to soothe their pain and discomfort?

Within a few minutes, the team brought this story to life, and the facilitators continued to invite the group to delve into the ramifications of events on the child's sense of self, trust in the world, and capacity to love other people. As a collective, the group inquired about the following: What do you think about this child and her experiences? Did anyone come when she cried? Did anyone touch her with compassion and care? Did anyone gaze into her eyes mirroring love? Eye gaze from birth onward activates the whole right side of the brain, including the empathy center, laying the groundwork for a safe relational template.[11]

Donna needed what she did not receive in her early years, beginning with soothing. Those close to her needed to help orient her to calm and soothing experiences in order to help fill the developmental gaps. This was not simply about correcting her overt challenging behaviors, but rather about starting the rebuild of her emotional world, her relational world in the brain, and the body to create a positive influence on her behavioral patterns.

With this understanding by her team, Donna was no longer classified as a child needing management or control. Rather she was considered a child that deserved attention, care, and connection. Now, rather than reacting to her challenging behaviors from fear-based brains, which lead to restraints, seclusion, and trying to use consequences to compel someone to behave better, her caregivers were able to care for her in an age-appropriate way that catered to her needs. Using a compassionate and relational perspective allowed an understanding of the developmental needs required for children to rebuild their foundation for emotional regulation and mutually enhancing relationships. Through the biographical timeline conversation, Donna was evaluated as a whole person. Being able to access compassionate curiosity helps individuals see themselves as social therapists who have the capacity to view daily life through a healing lens.

Through analysis of behaviors and interactions, the team realized Donna responded favorably to a deep touch and loved songs. Utilizing this knowledge, they were able to help her feel safe through positive touches and singing with her. This tactic was especially useful during bath time as the caregivers incorporated singing and soothing touches with the washcloth. Her caregivers would sing, "This is the way we wash your foot, wash your foot, wash your foot, this is the way we wash your foot, together in the evening." The songs oriented her to her body, offering safety, predictability, and the healing power of play.

Through this predictable, consistent, and safe routine, the team realized they were helping her integrate into her body. After a couple of weeks, she started to walk down the stairs without falling, and her bruises healed. Within months she no longer had tantrums, she would climb into her caregiver's lap to cuddle, and began to use more verbal language. Rather than "implementing a behavior plan," the team created predictability and consistency to enhance her capacity to feel safe with others.

Case Study 6-3

Eugene was a 16-year-old boy living a very isolated and painful life. At the time, he was nonverbal, self-abusive, and aggressive toward caregivers, especially women, often punching them when they would come too close. Staff in his residential facility were terrified of him, which led to restrictive procedures that meant he spent most of his time locked in his room, with a window in the door for observation purposes. The administration of the agency knew that this treatment could not continue, so they asked for a consultation. A team of social workers met with his team and anyone associated with Eugene currently and when possible, from his past in order to create a biographical timeline.

Discussion

Through the biographical timeline, the team learned that Eugene had been born in an understaffed orphanage in another country. Oftentimes the babies spent their beginning months living in tightly packed cribs with little human touch, eye contact, stimulation, or tenderness. After this traumatic start, he was placed in a home with an abusive foster mother. Subsequent placements were unsuccessful, as the caregivers, put off by his lack of engagement, isolating behaviors, and incessant rocking and crying, used increasingly punitive means to try to curb his behaviors. He was often scolded, spanked, and placed into timeout. When he reached adolescence, his behavior worsened, and he became more aggressive towards peers and caregivers. He was then placed in an institution to "contain his behaviors." When Eugene tried to communicate through gestures, the staff would not respond, because he was not using "real sign language." They did not want to feed into his "manipulative" behavior. While some of the staff had known that Eugene started his life in an orphanage that had a reputation for neglecting babies, they said, "Well, so what? That was a long time ago, there is no way that he could remember that and still be responding to his past experiences."

The facilitators used the opportunity afforded by the timeline to teach the staff members about developmental trauma and its long-term effects, as well as to remind them about the developmental attributes stemming from the vital exchange between an infant and their caregiver. The staff were then able to move into a compassionate space towards Eugene and eagerly strategized how they could work together to compensate for the "wounds, issues, and missed opportunities," employing their skills, talents, and passions on his behalf.

6 months later, Eugene could be found skateboarding with an exuberant staff person cheering him on. His team had engaged him in art, gardening, and craft work, and they had learned quite a few of his "signs" and now accepted his sign language. He in turn was starting to learn some of their more conventional signs as well.

KEY POINTS

1. When children are evaluated only by their overt challenging behaviors, punitive and pathologizing methods are often taken to manage and control the child's behaviors rather than address the root cause.

2. When punitive measures are taken, the child may continue to develop increasingly challenging behaviors and a distorted world view which exacerbates the problem.

3. Through the biographical timeline framework, someone can be understood more deeply, in the context of their life experiences, and compassionate supports that are relevant to the child can be built, leading to an enriched and emotionally healthy life, without the need to resort to challenging behaviors to have their needs met.

REFERENCES

1. Levine P, Kline M. *Trauma Through a Child's Eyes: Awakening the Ordinary Miracle of Healing.* North Atlantic Books; 2006.

2. Fisher SF. *Neurofeedback in the Treatment of Developmental Trauma: Calming the Fear-Driven Brain.* Norton and Company; 2014.

3. Collura TF, Siever D. Auditory-visual entrainment in relation to mental health and EEG. In: Budzynski TH, Budzynski HK, Evans JR, Abarbanel A, eds. *Introduction to Quantitative EEG and Neurofeedback: Advanced Theory and Applications.* 2nd ed. Academic Press; 2009:195-223.

4. Perry BD, Szalavitz M. *The Boy Who Was Raised as a Dog.* Basic Books; 2006.

5. Barol B. Revisiting the fourfold positive approaches paradigm: environment, communication, assessment, and hanging in there. *Pa J Posit Approach.* 2019;8(1):7-12.

6. Doidge N. *The Brain That Changes Itself: Stories of Personal Triumph from the Frontiers of Brain Science.* Penguin Random House; 2007.

7. van der Kolk B. *The Body Keeps the Score: Brain, Mind, and Body in the Healing of Trauma.* Penguin Random House; 2014.

8. Barol B. Learning from a person's biography: an introduction to the biographical timeline process. *Pa J Posit Approach.* 2001;3(4):20-29.

9. Jelley M, Wen F, Miller-Cribbs J, Coon K, Rodriguez K. Adverse childhood experiences, other psychosocial sources of adversity, and quality of life in vulnerable primary care patients. *Perm J.* 2020;24:18.277. doi:10.7812/TPP/18.277

10. Perry BD. Examining child maltreatment through a neurodevelopmental lens: clinical applications of the neurosequential model of therapeutics. *J Loss Trauma*. 2009;14(4):240-255. doi:10.1080/15325020903004350

11. Kochanska G, Boldt LJ, Goffin KC. Early relational experience: a foundation for the unfolding dynamics of parent–child socialization. *Child Dev Perspect*. 2019;13(1):41-47. doi:10.1111/cdep.12308

CLINICAL INTERVIEWING

Caitlin Rancher, PhD
Daniel W. Smith, PhD

OBJECTIVES
After reading this chapter, the reader will be able to:

1. *Describe the purpose of a clinical interview in the context of child exposure to trauma or maltreatment.*

2. *List specific strategies for conducting an effective clinical interview.*

3. *Prepare a comprehensive clinical interview that includes a detailed assessment of the identified traumatic event and a broad assessment of child functioning.*

BACKGROUND AND SIGNIFICANCE
Determining the need for treatment, establishing an accurate diagnosis, and providing evidence-based practice relies on information gathered during a clinical interview. Among children and adolescents who have experienced trauma or maltreatment, a comprehensive interview will include a broad assessment of the child's behavioral, social, and emotional functioning as well as a targeted focus on their experience of trauma and issues that may be related to the traumatic experience.

PURPOSE OF THE INTERVIEW
Prior to meeting with the child, the evaluator must be clear on the purpose of the clinical interview, especially in cases of child maltreatment. ***Clinical interviews*** are designed to assess a child's understanding of their experiences, explore the possible origin of symptoms, identify risk factors for serious problems, evaluate strengths and support, and guide further assessment and treatment. In contrast, a ***forensic interview*** is frequently used to determine whether a traumatic event occurred and to gather detailed information to support investigation or prosecution efforts. This is an important distinction, as clinical interviews typically include questions that, in a forensic context, would be considered "leading questions." The interviewer's mindset in a clinical interview is not oriented toward accuracy within legal rules of evidence, but toward accuracy in reflecting the child's psychological state and their needs. Clinical interviews include a broad assessment to inform whether and what type of treatment is appropriate for the child, regardless of whether the trauma allegations can be verified. This goal should be clearly communicated to the child and their caregivers as it can help set appropriate expectations and mitigate fears that the child will be judged or not believed.

INTERVIEW SOFT SKILLS
Clinical interviewing emphasizes face-to-face contact and interpersonal communication between the evaluator and the child. In successful clinical interviews, evaluators balance information gathering with effective communication and rapport. These "soft skills"—establishing and maintaining rapport; using unconditional positive regard and open body language; and encouraging engagement in the interview— are common to all clinical interviews and interventions.[1,2] Establishing trust and a

meaningful relationship with the child is critical to an effective interview. Children may fear the evaluator will judge them, not listen to or believe them, or be unable to tolerate hearing about their traumatic experience. Children may withhold information if they perceive the evaluator to be skeptical, judgmental, emotionally distressed, or easily shocked by offered information. Therefore, it is important for the evaluator to regulate their own responses to any disclosures made. The evaluator can provide appropriate validation and comfort with statements like, "Thank you for sharing that with me. That must have been a hard thing to do." These statements can help the child feel secure and listened to, and they can reduce fears of judgment or rejection. Other useful phrases to encourage the child to continue talking can include, "And then what happened?" or "Tell me more about that." The interviewer should avoid suggestive or critical questions such as, "Why didn't you ask them to stop?" or "Didn't you tell your mom about this?" These can be perceived as blaming the child for experiencing the traumatic event and may cause them to feel uncomfortable and withhold information.

BUILDING RAPPORT

Establishing comfortable and secure rapport is associated with higher quality clinical interview information.[3] Intentional, warm rapport building can help children feel more secure in the interview; this in turn can lead to them more readily sharing sensitive information. The developmental age of the child may determine the best way to build rapport. With young children, the evaluator may use common play or art activities to make the child feel more at ease and to facilitate communication. With older children, the evaluator may ask the child a few open-ended questions such as, "What do you know about coming to see me today?" or "What are you expecting to happen?" An evaluator may also begin the interview by asking about the child's interests or strengths with questions such as, "What do you like to do for fun?" or "What are some of the things you do really well?" These questions serve multiple purposes. For example:

— They can ease a child into the process of self-disclosure as they share information about themselves with the evaluator that is not related to trauma or maltreatment.

— They can provide clinical information on the child's strengths and assets that may inform treatment decisions.

— They can provide clinical insight into a child's self-perception, confidence, and social activities.

If a child provides negative responses such as, "I don't do anything well," this is useful information to incorporate into the conceptualization of the client. Maintaining rapport is an ongoing process throughout the clinical interview; however, the initial rapport-building stage should be brief—usually less than 8 minutes—to avoid cognitively exhausting the child or enabling avoidance of the more difficult topics that need to be assessed during the interview.[4]

CHALLENGES TO RAPPORT BUILDING

Evaluators may find it difficult to establish rapport with some children. Following trauma or maltreatment, children may feel nervous, scared, uncertain, angry, or any combination of these feelings when being asked questions by an unfamiliar adult. Some children may fear they will get in trouble or get someone they care about in trouble if they participate in the interview. Some children may feel overwhelmed by the process or frustrated at being asked what they perceive to be intrusive questions. Difficulty with rapport building can present heterogeneously: silence, denial (eg, "Nothing happened"), statements of ignorance (eg, "I don't know"), or attempts to distract the evaluator with play or by talking about other, unrelated topics. Unfortunately, there is no simple remedy for engaging children who are resistant to completing a clinical interview. However, the evaluator may employ various strategies depending on the individual child to get them more engaged. For example, for a fearful or overwhelmed child, the evaluator may engage them in more neutral topics or play a brief game to help them feel more secure and comfortable. The evaluator may reiterate the rationale for the interview to assuage fears of consequences or family trouble. The evaluator may validate the child's frustration by saying, "You are really feeling mad that your grandma brought you in here today." The evaluator may help keep the child focused by providing gentle redirection to the interview topics or allowing occasional breaks for play activities. Essentially, the evaluator must be flexible and meet the child—emotionally and developmentally—where they are when they attend the interview.

FLOW OF THE INTERVIEW

There are multiple ways to structure a clinical interview for a child who has experienced trauma or maltreatment. One comprehensive approach, adapted from the National Crime Victims Research & Treatment Center Family and Child Clinic at the Medical University of South Carolina, prioritizes collecting detailed information on the traumatic event and ensures broad assessment of the child's behavioral, social, and emotional functioning. There are no built-in breaks listed in this approach. The evaluator should use their clinical judgment to determine the pacing of the interview and provide appropriate breaks and encouragement, as needed.

PHASE 1: INTRODUCTION

During the introduction phase, the evaluator explains the goals of the clinical interview and establishes any ground rules. Exploring open-ended questions with the child about the purpose of the interview may be part of this phase. Typically, this is also the time when the evaluator will collect informed consent from the child's caregiver and assent from the child. As noted above, as part of the informed consent process, the evaluator should explain the differences between a clinical and forensic interview. The evaluator should then review confidentiality and its limits, with a particular focus on the need to report any new disclosures of child maltreatment or abuse discussed in the interview. Evaluators should also explain the flow and logistics of the interview, such as whether they will talk to the child alone or with a caregiver present. Taking extra time to address any of the child's questions or concerns will also help improve the quality of the interview.

PHASE 2: RAPPORT BUILDING

Rapport building allows the evaluator to establish an environment of trust where the child will feel comfortable answering questions. In addition to using open-ended questions to encourage self-disclosure on neutral or positive topics, the evaluator may also engage the child in a brief game or drawing activity. The goal of this phase is to help the child feel more secure and comfortable in the interview.

PHASE 3: TRAUMA ASSESSMENT

During the trauma assessment phase, the evaluator helps the child transition to the substantive portion of the interview. The goal of this phase is to conduct a detailed assessment of the presenting traumatic event and assess for the presence of any other trauma exposures. This broad assessment is critical as nearly 40% of children will experience multiple traumatic events in their lifetime.[5] Prematurely narrowing the focus of a clinical interview to a single identified traumatic event, even if it is the reason the child has been identified for services, risks overlooking important clinical information. The evaluator may start by asking broad questions such as, "Why do you think you were brought here today?" If the child does not mention any trauma experience, the evaluator should briefly share what they know about the child's trauma history and restate the purpose of the interview (eg, "My job is to find out more about what happened so that we can provide the best help possible"). The evaluator should then directly ask the child about different types of traumatic experiences. The evaluator can help provide rationale for this assessment by saying, "Stressful or scary events happen to many people; I want to know whether you have ever experienced…" A list of trauma experiences, including interpersonal violence, witnessing violence, non-interpersonal violence, and identity-based trauma, is presented in **Table 7-1.** This list is non-exhaustive, and the evaluator should follow up on other trauma experiences as needed. For young children or those with cognitive or developmental disabilities, the evaluator may conduct this detailed assessment of trauma experiences with the child's caregiver.

Table 7-1. Trauma Experiences to Assess for in Clinical Interview

Type of Trauma	Example
Interpersonal Violence or Maltreatment	— Robbed by threat, force, or weapon
	— Slapped, punched, or beat up by someone in your family
	— Slapped, punched, or beat up by someone not in your family
	— Someone older touching your private parts when they shouldn't
	— Someone forcing or pressuring sex, or when you couldn't say no
	— Attacked, stabbed, shot at, or hurt badly
	— Had peers threaten, make fun of, or spread rumors about you
	— Times when you did not have enough to eat, have clothing, or a safe place to sleep
	— Times when you did not receive help that you needed from a doctor
	— Times when an adult said insulting or mean things to put you down or make you feel bad
Witnessing Family Violence	— Seeing someone in your family get slapped, punched, or beat up
	— Seeing someone in your family attacked, stabbed, shot at, hurt badly, or killed
Witnessing Community Violence in Real Life (not in media)	— Seeing someone in the community get slapped, punched, or beat up
	— Seeing someone in the community attacked, stabbed, shot at, hurt badly, or killed
	— Being around war
Non-Interpersonal Violence or Trauma	— Serious natural disasters like floods, tornadoes, hurricanes, earthquakes, or fires
	— Serious accident or injury like a car/bike crash or sports injury
	— Someone close to you dying suddenly or violently
	— Someone close to you experiencing a sudden, serious illness
	— Stressful or scary medical procedure
Identity-Based Trauma	— Discrimination based on your gender, race, ethnicity, sexual orientation, religion/spirituality, or other part of your identity
	— Discrimination or prejudice based on your skin color, where you or your family were born, or the language you speak

Note. This table provides a non-exhaustive list of trauma experiences to assess for in a clinical interview among children who have experienced trauma or maltreatment.

The evaluator should then conduct a thorough assessment about the traumatic event(s) the child disclosed—how often it occurred, where it took place, when it began, when it ended, who was involved, how it was discovered, how caregivers and guardians responded, and whether the event was reported to any authorities or agencies. In the event the child's trauma involves a series of traumatic events (eg, chronic sexual or physical abuse) or the child discloses multiple traumatic events, the evaluator should prioritize gathering information on the most distressing event but may also include the first and most recent events. For many children, the first traumatic event may have been the most surprising—challenging previously held worldviews about safety and trust. In some cases, the first traumatic event may not have previously been disclosed to caregivers or authorities. The evaluator should be familiar with the professional, ethical, and legal standards for reporting child abuse in the state in which they are practicing. As noted above, the evaluator should also prepare children and their families during the introduction phase about when a mandated report to authorities might be necessary. There is also value in assessing the details of the most recent event. Frequently, this is the traumatic experience that led to the disclosure or discovery of child maltreatment or abuse. The most recent event may be having the most immediate effect on child functioning at the time of the clinical interview.

PHASE 4: TRAUMA SYMPTOMS

The trauma symptoms phase involves a narrowed focus on the primary symptoms and impairment the child is experiencing as a result of the trauma. The evaluator should utilize the child's language to describe the traumatic event. The evaluator may use open-ended questions such as, "What kinds of changes in your life have you noticed since (trauma) occurred?" or "How has (trauma) been affecting your life?" The evaluator should seek to establish whether these problems were present before the traumatic event occurred or whether functioning has changed since the event. The evaluator may consider supplementing their clinical interview with a standardized assessment measure of trauma symptoms. Many self-report assessments can facilitate comparison of the child's symptoms to clinical norms, which can be useful in determining the degree of impairment. They can also provide the basis for more specific follow-up questions about endorsed symptoms. For example, the evaluator could reflect, "You selected 'Almost Always' for trying to avoid places, people, or things that remind you of the (trauma). Tell me more about that." It is important for the evaluator to recognize that many children who experience a traumatic event exhibit considerable resilience, and not all will go on to experience significant psychological distress or impairment.[6-8] Additionally, some children may be experiencing psychological distress or impairment unrelated to the traumatic event. The goal of this phase is to establish a functional relation between the trauma exposure and reported symptoms to best inform whether the child would benefit from trauma-focused treatment. Functional relations can be difficult to determine with certainty, but they can be established with reasonable confidence by identifying temporal associations between traumatic events and symptoms, or by a logical relationship between the trauma and the symptom (eg, nightmares about the event or distress over situations that are similar to the trauma).

PHASE 5: ADDITIONAL SYMPTOMS

During the fifth phase, the evaluator explores additional areas of distress or impairment. It is critical for evaluators to include a broad assessment of psychological distress, as past research has consistently shown that trauma symptoms are highly comorbid with other internalizing and externalizing problems.[9] The additional clinical interview questions can be guided by standardized assessment measures completed by either the child, caregiver, or both. Common areas to assess include depression, anxiety, psychosis, sleep disturbances, behavior problems, and substance use. Asking caregivers and children to complete standardized assessment measures prior to the interview allows the evaluator to focus on additional symptoms causing the most distress or impairment. However, the evaluator should not limit their interview to symptoms reported on the assessment measures. The interview should include a broad exploration of symptoms. The evaluator may begin this phase by asking, "What other problems have you noticed?" or "What other difficulties are you having at home or school?" The evaluator should follow these inquiries with specific questions assessing for details (eg, frequency, severity) of any endorsed symptoms.

PHASE 6: COPING SKILLS

During the coping skills phase, clinicians should seek detailed clinical information on the strategies—positive and negative—the child has been using to manage their distress. The evaluator may ask the child, "What do you do when you are feeling upset?" with specific follow-up questions related to "What has worked best for you?" or "What have you tried that didn't work?" Assessing existing coping strategies helps inform treatment planning. For example, if a child endorses using deep breathing or relaxation skills, this may be a strength that is built into their treatment. Children may also endorse maladaptive or ineffective strategies such as avoidance, self-harm, aggression, or substance use. This also provides useful insight to inform treatment planning and case conceptualization. When the child discloses a maladaptive coping strategy, the evaluator should recall the goals of the clinical interview—this is not the time to challenge or criticize a child's behavior. Nevertheless, if the child does disclose risky or dangerous behavior, the evaluator may need to conduct a risk assessment and create a safety plan.

PHASE 7: SAFETY ASSESSMENT

The safety assessment is the phase of the interview where safety plans are created if risky or dangerous behavior has been disclosed. There is a detailed focus on suicidality, self-harm, and risk assessment. Recent meta-analyses have found that trauma symptoms are associated with increased incidence of past suicide attempts and current suicidal ideation.[10] The evaluator may focus on interview questions that screen for suicidality such as, "Have you wished you were dead or wished you could go to sleep and not wake up?" or "Have you had any thoughts of killing yourself?" If positively endorsed, these questions should be followed by a detailed interview to assess for plan, intent, lethality, and access to lethal means. The evaluator should be prepared to respond to any disclosed safety concerns, including but not limited to completing a safety plan, informing the child's caregiver, and navigating possible inpatient hospitalization.

PHASE 8: SOCIAL AND ACADEMIC HISTORY

The social and academic history phase is an exploration of the child's broader social environment, relationships, and academic performance. In a recent meta-analysis of protective factors following children's exposure to violence, Yule and colleagues[11] found that family support, peer support, and school support were critical predictors of children's recovery from trauma and violence. Thus, a thorough understanding of a child's home and school environment and their relationships with caregivers and peers has important implications for their recovery and treatment plan. The evaluator may provide a brief rationale (ie, "An important part of getting to know you is learning about your family and school") and ask broad questions such as, "What is it like growing up in your family?" or "How do you get along with your caregivers?" The evaluator should include interview questions regarding peer relationships—both platonic and romantic—as well as questions on the child's school performance. Information on behavior problems at school, special accommodations, and relationships with teachers can all provide insight into the child's broader ecological context.

The evaluator can also use this phase to explore the child's identity and cultural background in greater depth. The evaluator can explain this section by saying something similar to the following:

I'd like to ask you a few additional questions to learn more about you, your caregiver, and your family's identity. We know that parts of one's personal identity and cultural background can have an important influence on their wellbeing, views, and response to treatment.

The evaluator may combine broad open-ended questions such as, "What parts of your background or identity would be important for me to understand?" as well as specific questions about the child's identity. The evaluator may include questions related to other's reactions to an aspect of the child's identity, how it has affected the child, and how their experience of their identity influences their understanding of their trauma experience. The evaluator should keep the child's cognitive and developmental abilities in mind; in general, older children and adolescents are more likely to be able to provide insight and detailed responses to questions about their identity. For detailed discussion on the effects of child maltreatment and trauma across specific groups and identities (eg, children with disabilities, LGBTQIA+ children), see Volume 2, Section II: Intersectional Considerations and Applications.

Phase 9: Child's Goals

The final phase of the interview is focused on exploring the child's goals for therapy. The evaluator may ask, "What are the 3 major goals you have for therapy?" or "What are the 3 most important issues for us to address?" These questions help instill hope that relief from distressing symptoms is possible. These questions also afford the child some autonomy in defining what they see as most important to focus on in treatment. It is not uncommon for younger children to not have any goals for therapy, and so these questions may be more appropriate to address with the child's caregiver. At the end of the interview, the evaluator should ask the child whether they have anything else they would like to disclose.

Sensitivity to Diversity

Effective clinical interviewing involves attention and sensitivity to diversity. Previous research has found that, compared to White individuals, those who are considered racial and ethnic minorities are less likely to engage in mental health treatment, feel less satisfied with mental health services, and are more likely to drop out from treatment prematurely.[12] The systemic issues perpetuating these disparities are complex; however, evaluators can take special care during a clinical interview to help all children feel more understood and engaged. The evaluator should be mindful of the client's multicultural identity and need for cultural competence throughout the interview. As detailed above, this includes careful assessment of the child's identity and how their identity informs or has influenced their experience of trauma. The evaluator should ask questions to better understand the child and their family's perspective. This may include asking about a caregiver or family member's reactions to the traumatic event such as, "Does your family see what happened as a 'private matter?'" or "Does your family see what happened as something to be ashamed of?" If the child experienced the sudden or violent loss of a loved one, then the evaluator should take extra time to understand the child's religious and spiritual beliefs, including what the child believes happens when people die. Although many evaluators express reservations or discomfort in assessing and discussing religion and spirituality, it is important to consider that many clients express a desire for their beliefs—and all aspects of their identity—to be addressed in treatment.[13]

Case Study

Case Study 7-1

A 9-year-old girl presented to a mental health clinic following a recent disclosure of sexual abuse allegedly perpetrated by her soccer coach. The parents reported that she has been having nightmares, seems distracted, and has been fighting at school. The parents asked their daughter about her behavior, and she disclosed the abuse. The parents contacted law enforcement. After conducting a forensic assessment, the police recommended a clinical evaluation. The assigned therapist interviewed the child to help understand how her experiences might be functionally related to her symptoms. The therapist assessed multiple different traumatic experiences and learned the child had also experienced physically abusive punishment from an uncle who used to live in the home. The clinical interview determined her symptoms were related to her experiences of sexual and physical abuse. The child's symptoms, strengths, and coping skills were all considered in recommending trauma-focused treatment.

Discussion

The child was referred based on a confirmed report of one type of maltreatment. However, a thorough trauma screen revealed an additional form of abuse that was also contributing to the clinical presentation. Had the therapist not completed a broader trauma assessment, a key contributing factor to her symptoms would have gone undetected. This newly disclosed physical abuse will require the therapist to make a supplemental mandated report.

KEY POINTS

1. The goal of a clinical interview is to inform whether and what type of treatment is appropriate for a child who has experienced trauma or maltreatment.

2. A comprehensive clinical interview will include a detailed assessment of the identified traumatic event and other possible trauma exposures as well as a broad assessment of the child's behavioral, social, and emotional functioning.

3. Establishing a comfortable rapport and attending to the client's multicultural identity are critical for conducting a quality clinical interview.

REFERENCES

1. Akseer R, Connolly M, Cosby J, Frost G, Kanagarajah RR, Lim SE. Clinician-patient relationships after two decades of a paradigm of patient-centered care. *Int J Healthc Manag.* 2020;1-10. doi:10.1080/ 20479700.2020.1713535

2. Sburlati ES, Schniering CA, Lyneham HJ, Rapee RM. A model of therapist competencies for the empirically supported cognitive behavioral treatment of child and adolescent anxiety and depressive disorders. *Clin Child Fam Psychol Rev.* 2011;14(1):89-109. doi:10.1007/s10567-011-0083-6

3. DeJonckheere M, Vaughn LM. Semistructured interviewing in primary care research: A balance of relationship and rigour. *J Fam Med Community Health.* 2019;7(2):1-8. doi:10.1136/fmch-2018-000057

4. Saywitz KL, Larson RP, Hobbs SD, Wells CR. Developing rapport with children in forensic interviews: systematic review of experimental research. *Behav Sci Law.* 2015;33(4):372-390. doi:10.1002/bsl.2186

5. Le MT, Holton S, Romero L, Fisher J. Polyvictimization among children and adolescents in low- and lower-middle-income countries: A systematic review and meta-analysis. *Trauma Violence Abuse.* 2018;19(3):323-42. doi:10.1177/ 1524838016659489

6. Andrews AR, Jobe-Shields L, López CM, et al. Polyvictimization, income, and ethnic differences in trauma-related mental health during adolescence. *Soc Psychiatry Psychiatr Epidemiol.* 2015;50(8):1223-1234. doi:10.1007/s00127-015-1077-3

7. Gren-Landell M, Aho N, Andersson G, Svedin CG. Social anxiety disorder and victimization in a community sample of adolescents. *J Adolesc.* 2011;34(3):569-577. doi:10.1016/j.adolescence.2010.03.007

8. Turner HA, Finkelhor D, Ormrod R, et al. Family context, victimization, and child trauma symptoms: variations in safe, stable, and nurturing relationships

during early and middle childhood. *Am J Orthopsychiatry.* 2012;82(2):209-219. doi:10.1111/j.1939-0025.2012.01147.x

9. De Young AC, Kenardy JA, Cobham VE. Trauma in early childhood: A neglected population. *Clin Child Fam Psychol Rev.* 2011;14(3):231-50. doi:10.1007/s10567-011-0094-3

10. Krysinska K, Lester D. Post-traumatic stress disorder and suicide risk: a systematic review. *Arch Suicide Res.* 2010;14(1):1-23. doi:10.1080/13811110903478997

11. Yule K, Houston J, Grych J. Resilience in children exposed to violence: A meta-analysis of protective factors across ecological contexts. *Clin Child Fam Psychol Rev.* 2019;22(3):406-31. doi:10.1007/s10567-019-00293-1

12. Maura J, Weisman de Mamani A. Mental health disparities, treatment engagement, and attrition among racial/ethnic minorities with severe mental illness: A review. *J Clin Psychol Med Settings.* 2017;24(3):187-210. doi:10.1007/s10880-017-9510-2

13. Harris KA, Randolph BE, Gordon TD. What do clients want? Assessing spiritual needs in counseling: A literature review. *Spiritual Clin Pract.* 2016;3(4):250-275. doi:10.1037/scp0000108

Preschool Assessment

Alytia Levendosky, PhD
Lia Field Martin, PhD
Alexandra L. Ballinger, MA

Objectives
After reading this chapter, the reader will be able to:

1. *Recognize the various developmental systems affected by child maltreatment in preschool-age children.*

2. *Identify appropriate clinical assessment tools for use in this population.*

3. *Describe the clinical diagnoses common in maltreated preschool-age children.*

Background and Significance

The Children's Bureau of the United States Department of Health and Human Services' Child Maltreatment 2020 Report[1] indicated that rates of preschool children who experience maltreatment are about 9 in every 1000, which is lower than infants but higher than older children. Additionally, larger political and contextual events cause rates of childhood maltreatment to vary. For example, during 2020-2021, the height of COVID-19, increases in economic hardship and social isolation had significant concurrent increases in the frequency and severity of child abuse cases.[2,3]

Child maltreatment does not usually result in a single, well defined set of symptoms such as increased anxiety or mood problems; rather, maltreatment often results in diffuse, wide-ranging impairment.[4,5] More specifically, maltreatment exposure during the first 5 years of life has disruptive, cascading effects across multiple domains that are undergoing rapid and significant development in these years. A commonly used framework to account for this diffuse impairment is Developmental Trauma Disorder (DTD),[6] which is currently only a proposed diagnosis. However, this framework is considered useful in that it includes the developmental disruptions across the following domains of functioning: attachment; biological, affective, and behavioral regulation; and cognitive functioning.

Attachment

An essential task of early childhood is the development of an attachment to a primary caregiver or caregivers. Attachment refers to the affective bond between a child and caregiver that serves to promote proximity and to protect the child in circumstances of threat or danger.[7] The attachment bond is developed over repeated caregiving interactions. When caregivers reliably meet a child's needs, the child learns they are safe to freely explore their environment and seek support if needed, confident that they will be cared for and protected.[7]

Individual differences in attachment are present by 1 year of age, and the organization of children's attachment depends on the quality of the caregiving they receive. Children's attachment is categorized into 4 types based on the behaviors they exhibit when separated from their primary caregiver: secure, avoidant, ambivalent, and disorganized.[8] Children with **secure attachment** are confident in their caregiver's availability and responsiveness and freely seek comfort from them. Children with *avoidant attachment* expect rejection from their caregiver and do not seek comfort from them. Children with *ambivalent attachment* are unsure about the responsiveness of their caregiver and both seek and resist comfort from them. Finally, children with *disorganized attachment* display confused, bizarre behavior and lack a coherent attachment strategy.

When perpetrated by a parent or caregiver, maltreatment becomes an attachment trauma. Maltreatment severely dysregulates the child's attachment system and undermines their confidence in the safety of their caregivers. These experiences cause children to develop more negative representations of their caregivers, themselves, and the caregiver-child relationship.[9] Maltreated children are less likely to develop secure attachment but are more likely to exhibit disorganized attachment even when compared with children experiencing other sociodemographic risk factors.[10] Maltreating parents may disorganize their children's attachment system because they are paradoxically both a source of comfort and a threat, causing the child's approach and avoidance impulses to be in conflict.[10] Attachment disorganization predisposes children to future interpersonal problems and psychopathology.[11] There are various parent-report questionnaire assessments of attachment in preschool children that can be used by clinicians as seen in **Table 8-1.**

Table 8-1. Parent-Report Questionnaires of Attachment in Preschool Children	
QUESTIONNAIRE ASSESSMENT NAME	DESCRIPTION
Mothers' Object Relations Scale[12]	14-item scale assessing mother's internal representations of their child. For ages 2 to 4 years.
Child-Parent Relationship Scale[13]	30 or 15 (short form) item measure of parents' views of their relationship with their child. For ages 3 years and older.
Parenting Stress Index[14]	120 or 36 (short form) item measure of parenting stress including parents' views and expectations of their child. For ages 0 to 12 years.

BIOLOGICAL REGULATION

Biological systems and internal regulation are also affected by maltreatment. *Biological regulation* refers to the body's capacity to adjust biological functions to maintain internal homeostasis.[15] Stress response systems, particularly the sympathetic nervous system (SNS) and the hypothalamic-pituitary-adrenal (HPA) axis, are most impacted by maltreatment.[16,17] When an individual encounters a stressor, the SNS (ie, the fight or flight response) mobilizes to help the individual flee or confront the threat. Subsequently, the HPA axis is activated and secretes the stress hormone cortisol.[15] Timely activation and deactivation of the stress response system is critical for adaptive functioning.

However, chronic SNS and HPA axis activation due to repeated stressors, such as recurring child maltreatment, can become pathogenic. HPA axis alterations can result in *hypercortisolism* (ie, an excess of circulating cortisol) or *hypocortisolism* (ie, reduced levels of cortisol). Both of these conditions can result in an inability to respond appropriately to stressors.[16] Hypocortisolism in particular is thought to occur after repeated exposure to interpersonal trauma, such as child maltreatment. One meta-analysis[17] found blunted stress reactivity in individuals of all ages following exposure to child maltreatment, while another[18] reported blunted wakening cortisol levels in children with substantiated maltreatment histories. Furthermore, an additional meta-analysis[16] reported blunted cardiovascular reactivity in general—and blunted SNS reactivity specifically—in maltreated children.

The HPA axis has important regulatory effects on sleep, obesity, mental illness, and physical health.[19,20] Therefore, dysregulation of the HPA axis impacts biological systems regulated by diurnal cortisol patterns. For instance, flattened diurnal cortisol is associated with sleep disruption, overeating/obesity, and externalizing behavior problems in children.[21] Diurnal cortisol dysregulation likely contributes to the increased rates of sleep disturbances, emotion dysregulation, and behavioral problems observed in maltreated preschoolers.[20] While it is not practical to directly assess children's biological regulation in clinical practice, behavioral manifestations of the underlying biological systems can be measured using various assessment tools.

AFFECTIVE AND BEHAVIORAL REGULATION

Dysregulation of biological systems can also contribute to problems with affective, emotional, and behavioral regulation in maltreated children. ***Emotional regulation*** is broadly defined as the capacity to initiate, inhibit, or adjust the expression of internal emotional states and their associated behaviors in terms of duration and intensity.[5] Maltreated preschool children show deficits in emotional regulation.[5,22]

During the first 3 years of life, a child primarily relies on caregivers for assistance with regulation, often called coregulation.[23] In these early years, experiences with their parents shape children's self-regulatory capacities and entrain functionality to self-regulate in times of distress.[24] When a child's emotional coregulation is suboptimal (eg, due to child maltreatment), their self-regulatory capacity may be deficient, which becomes the precursor for subsequent psychopathology.[23] Between the ages of 3 and 5, children develop increased capacity for independent emotional regulation, so early signs of psychopathology often manifest during this time.[24]

Maltreating parents are often poor models of appropriate emotional self-regulation. They typically are not effective at coregulating their children and may respond to their children's emotional behavior with aggression, hostility,[25] or intrusive or controlling behavior.[26] These parents may also respond to their children's emotional arousal in invalidating or dismissive ways, or they may fail to provide any meaningful response altogether.[26] Finally, maltreating parents tend to be less sensitive to their young children's emotional experiences. Research has shown that parents' inability to teach their children strategies for emotion regulation, when also coupled with their lack of sensitivity, directly explains why maltreated children lack the capacity to effectively manage their emotional arousal.[27]

Particularly among preschoolers, there are significant pattern differences of emotion regulation between maltreated and non-maltreated children when exposed to arousing situations.[28] Maltreated children are typically highly attuned to anger; they are able to perceive anger with far fewer cues than non-maltreated children, which is understood to be an adaptation to a threatening environment.[29] Deficits in emotion regulation among preschool-age children might be expressed as internalizing behaviors (eg, depression, anxiety, somatic disorders) or externalizing behaviors (eg, attention deficits, aggression, defiance), both of which can increase across childhood.[30,31]

An assessment of emotional and behavioral regulation is most effectively done with parent report questionnaires (see **Table 8-2**).

Table 8-2. Parent-Report Questionnaires of Affective/Behavioral Regulation in Preschool Children	
QUESTIONNAIRE ASSESSMENT NAME	DESCRIPTION
Brief Infant-Toddler Social and Emotional Assessment[32]	42-item measure of problems and competence in the affective/behavioral realm. For ages 1 to 3 years.

(continued)

Table 8-2. Parent-Report Questionnaires of Affective/Behavioral Regulation in Preschool Children *(continued)*

QUESTIONNAIRE ASSESSMENT NAME	DESCRIPTION
Child Behavior Checklist[33]	100-item questionnaire of internalizing and externalizing broad-band scales, as well as narrow scales of attention problems, somatic complaints, and anxiety/depression, among others. For ages 1 1/2 to 5 years.
The Behavior Assessment System for Children, 3rd Edition[34]	139-item assessment tool of emotional and behavioral strengths and weaknesses. For ages 2 to 5 years. This assessment also has a 105-item assessment tool for teachers.

COGNITIVE DISRUPTIONS AND IMPAIRED EXECUTIVE FUNCTIONING

Early childhood maltreatment has deleterious effects on children's cognitive development.[35] Early maltreatment, especially neglect, is associated with cognitive delays for a number of years after the substantiated maltreatment,[36] and it may negatively impact later intellectual functioning, particularly verbal comprehension and processing speed.[37]

In addition to intellectual abilities, executive function (EF) may be disrupted due to early childhood maltreatment. Broadly explained, EF is comprised of all abilities necessary to effectively organize one's goal-directed behavior. EF includes the ability to shift attention between stimuli, respond quickly and flexibly to new information, hold and manipulate information in one's mind, and understand the consequences of one's actions.[38] Two subdomains of EF in particular are negatively impacted by early childhood maltreatment: attentional control (ie, the ability to intentionally focus attention on a task or object while also ignoring nonessential information) and working memory (ie, the ability to hold information in mind for a brief time, and being able to readily access and manipulate it).[38,39] Maltreated preschoolers attend differently to expressions of emotion, with an attentional bias toward threat-related cues (eg, angry faces),[29,40] indicative of vigilance toward future harm. Anxiously attending to potential threats in their environment may be adaptive in the short-term for maltreated children; however, sustained attention to threats over an extended period of time may result in later difficulties with self-regulation and interpersonal skills as a result of frequently perceiving a threat where none exists.[29,40]

Research has also found a link between maltreatment and other aspects of EF in preschool-age children, including spatial working memory (measured at 26 months of age)[41] and inhibitory control (ie, the ability to override a dominant or habitual response in favor of a response that is more goal-directed).[40,42] The early cognitive impairment observed in these children is also predictive of learning and academic difficulties later in life, such as decreased attentional control, which may result in them being unable to process academic material adequately.[43] Additionally, EF is essential for adaptive functioning, which refers to a wide set of learned abilities comprised of three domains: social skills (eg, social imitation, initiation of joint play), communication skills (eg, language use), and practical daily life skills (eg, getting dressed, using the bathroom independently, motor skills such as cutting and gluing). Children with trauma histories demonstrate poorer adaptive function in all three domains, with chronic neglect exerting the most negative impact.[44] One study found that maltreated children demonstrate an average discrepancy of 5 years between chronological and developmental age for adaptive functioning skills.[45] In sum, the cognitive impact of early childhood maltreatment has important implications for children's psychosocial functioning both within and outside of the classroom (see **Table 8-3**).

Table 8-3. Assessments of Cognitive and Executive Functioning in Preschool Children

QUESTIONNAIRE ASSESSMENT NAME	DESCRIPTION
Wechsler Preschool and Primary Scale of Intelligence[46]	A comprehensive standardized set of tasks and questions that assess general intellectual ability as well as domains of cognition, such as how quickly a child can process information, reasoning and comprehension skills, knowledge acquisition, and receptive and expressive language skills. For ages 2 to 7 years.
Stanford-Binet Intelligence Scales for Early Childhood[47]	A comprehensive standardized set of tasks and questions that assess overall intellectual ability as well as domains of cognition such as speed of information processing, memory, reasoning and comprehension, knowledge acquisition, and receptive and expressive language skills. For ages 2 to 5 years.
The NEPSY-II[48]	A standardized set of 32 neuropsychological tasks that assess memory, attention, sensorimotor functioning, learning, social-emotional perception, planning, flexibility in thinking, language, and communication. For ages 3 to 16 years.
The Behavior Rating Inventory of Executive Function- Preschool version[49]	A 63-item survey in which caregivers report on a child's executive functioning skills as they appear in their daily home and school environments. For ages 2 to 5 years.
Conners Kiddie Continuous Performance Test[50]	A 7.5-minute-long test given on a computer screen. Children are shown images of target and non-target items. Children are instructed to hit a key when they see target images and inhibit response to non-targets. It assesses their signal detection, response time, and inhibition. For ages 4 to 7 years.
The Vineland Adaptive Behavior Scales Third Edition (VABS-3)[51]	A standardized semi-structured interview tool for assessing developmental delays and adaptive behavior, including social relationships, communication, and activities of daily living. Parent version for ages 0 to 90+ years; teacher version for ages 3 to 21 years.

DISSOCIATION

Another symptom commonly experienced by maltreated children and related to EF is *dissociation*, defined as a lack of integration between sensory and perception systems, attention, and memory. Clinically, dissociation can manifest as trance-like states, problems with autobiographical memory, rapidly fluctuating and intense mood states, belief in alternative selves or imaginary friends, derealization, and depersonalization.[52] While low levels of dissociative experiences (eg, frequent day-dreaming) are normative in childhood, maltreated children are at an increased risk of pathological levels of dissociation, which can lead to significant impairments in functioning, a fragmented sense of self-identity, memory disturbances, and impaired attention.[36,53,54] Children who experience high levels of dissociation may become confused and unable to recall important events that have happened. These children may also exhibit rapid changes in their feelings and behavior, and they may have difficulty maintaining a cohesive sense of self.[52,54] While all types of child maltreatment are associated with dissociative symptoms, the most profound dissociation appears to be associated with physical abuse and physical abuse co-occurring with neglect.[53]

Assessing dissociation in preschool-age children can be challenging, given that some normative psychological phenomena observed at this age, such as having imaginary friends, confusion in temporal memory (eg, mixing up tomorrow and yesterday), or absorption in fantasy play, can also be indicative of emerging dissociative processes. Clinical assessment parent-report tools can help differentiate between normative and clinically elevated forms of dissociation (see **Table 8-4**).

Table 8-4. Parent-Report Questionnaires of Affective/Behavioral Regulation in Preschool Children	
QUESTIONNAIRE ASSESSMENT NAME	DESCRIPTION
Child Dissociative Checklist[55]	20-item questionnaire for caregivers that assesses behavioral indicators of dissociation in children. For ages 5 to 12 years.
Trauma Symptom Checklist for Young Children[56]	90-item questionnaire for parents, including a specific scale for dissociation. For ages 3 to 17 years.

CLINICAL DISORDERS

Due to the damaging effects of child maltreatment across multiple domains of functioning, it is unsurprising that maltreated children are 3 times more likely than non-maltreated children to develop mental health disorders.[57,58] Specifically, in terms of internalizing disorders, a large meta-analysis of children and adolescents in the welfare system[57] found that about 11% of this population develop depression and 18% develop an anxiety disorder during childhood. Rates of externalizing disorders were also high, including ADHD (11%), oppositional defiant disorder (12%), and conduct disorder (20%).[57]

The mood, anxiety, and behavioral disorders noted above are all observed in higher rates in maltreated children, but they are not specific to abused children. Conversely, *reactive attachment disorder* (RAD) is an emotional disturbance that occurs only in maltreated children.[59] The core feature of RAD is a pattern of inappropriate social relations, characterized by a persistent reluctance to initiate relationships or to accept affection from even familiar adults or caregivers. On the other end of the spectrum, children with RAD can also display an excessive need to solicit affection from any available adult, even those with whom they are not familiar.[60] Additionally, regulatory disorders are more likely to be seen in maltreated than non-maltreated preschoolers. These disorders are characterized by poorly modulated patterns of sleeping, eating, or elimination; problems with fine or gross motor skills; and sensory integration problems.[61] Children with regulatory problems can also appear either hypersensitive or hyposensitive to physical touch, loud noises, or bright lights.[61]

Finally, one of the most common disturbances associated with child maltreatment is post-traumatic stress disorder (PTSD). One meta-analysis found that rates of PTSD in maltreated boys are about 17%, and in maltreated girls, the rate is about 32%.[62] However, these prevalence rates are based on adult-oriented *Diagnostic and Statistical Manual of Mental Disorders* (DSM) criteria, and young children tend not to meet these criteria even when exposed to trauma.[63] In response to this problem, the fifth edition of the *Diagnostic and Statistical Manual of Mental Disorders* (DSM-5) has modified the PTSD diagnostic criteria for children 6 years old and younger. However, one study[64] found that this modification is still not a good fit for the trauma symptoms evident in young children. Instead, the developmentally sensitive criteria in DC:0-5[61] for PTSD is the best diagnostic criteria to use for young children experiencing maltreatment as of the writing of this chapter.

Assessment of maltreatment and associated psychopathology in preschool-age children should be done considering the full context of the child's experience and cultural factors, and multiple informants should be used to gain the best understanding of the child's experience. The National Child Traumatic Stress Network[65] has resources to assist clinicians in screening, assessing, and treating childhood traumatic sequelae (see **Table 8-5**).

Table 8-5. Parent-Report Questionnaires of PTSD and Related Disorders in Preschool Children	
ASSESSMENT NAME	DESCRIPTION
Traumatic Events Screening Inventory[66]	24-item questionnaire for parents, assessing exposure to potentially traumatic events. For ages 4 to 18.
Trauma Symptom Checklist for Young Children[56]	90-item questionnaire for parents, yielding scores for symptoms such as PTSD, depression, and anger. For ages 3 to 12.
Clinician Administered Diagnostic Infant and Preschool Assessment[67]	Structured clinical interview with parents that yields diagnoses, including PTSD and reactive attachment disorder, among others. For ages 0 to 6.

CONCLUSION

It is evident that preschool-age children who experience child maltreatment show negative effects across multiple domains of functioning, consistent with the DTD model of effects of interpersonal trauma. Thus, assessments for children who have experienced child maltreatment should cover the breadth of domains of functioning, as discussed above, rather than limiting assessments to clinical disorders commonly associated with maltreatment, such as RAD or PTSD. A full battery of assessments that cover all of these domains of functioning will be better able to inform treatment. Finally, due to deficits across domains of functioning for preschool-age children who experienced maltreatment, evidence-based treatments should focus on the parent-child system and the systemic effects on development.

CASE STUDY

Case Study 8-1

Sally and Robert, twins, entered treatment when they were 5 years old. They had suffered physical abuse as well as physical and emotional neglect from their parents, and had witnessed IPV since they were born. At the age of 4 1/2 years, they were legally removed from their parents and placed in the custody of their paternal grandparents. The grandparents reported having discovered their grandchildren as toddlers locked in a room by themselves for hours at a time with no food or water, while their parents were unconscious in the living room after drug use. They discovered their grandchildren at least 3 times in this situation, each time resulting in them taking the children for a couple of months, but returning them again to their home upon the parents' entreaties until a judge ordered the children to be removed from parental custody. The grandparents also reported that the children had witnessed violence between their parents, as well as aggressive sexual behavior between a variety of adults. Finally, they reported that the parents frequently alternated between hostile, angry behavior and neglectful, uninterested behavior with regards to the twins, often not holding them or touching them for days.

Discussion

Due to the extensive experiences of multiple forms of maltreatment experienced by these children, assessment across multiple domains of functioning is warranted. First, an assessment of each child's attachment is important as well as the parenting stress likely experienced by the grandparents who were not expecting to parent their grandchildren full-time. These assessments will help the clinician understand the effects of the maltreatment on the children's attachment styles and also likely intervention for both the children and their grandparents. Second, assessment of each child's affective and behavioral regulation is essential for guiding treatment. This should be assessed with the grandparents through interviews as well as the use of a standardized questionnaire. Finally, assessment of traumatic and dissociative symptoms is also essential here due to the severity of the abuse and neglect. This can be done using standardized questionnaires or interviews with the grandparents. Taken together, these assessments will inform case conceptualization for each of the twins and guide child therapy as well as any potential parent work or family therapy to support the grandparents in their new parenting roles.

KEY POINTS

1. Child maltreatment leads to damage in multiple domains of functioning; thus, the DTD framework is a helpful approach.

2. Clinical tools that assess children's multiple domains of functioning and help screen for mental disorders are important for understanding the full range of the effects of maltreatment.

3. Treatments should focus on the parent-child system in order to create safety for the child and allow them to resume normal developmental functioning.

REFERENCES

1. US Department of Health and Human Services; Administration for Children and Families. Child Maltreatment 2020. 2022. https://www.acf.hhs.gov/sites/default/files/documents/cb/cm2020.pdf

2. Swedo E, Idaikkadar N, Leemis R, et al. Trends in US emergency department visits related to suspected or confirmed child abuse and neglect among children and adolescents aged <18 years before and during the Covid-19 pandemic — United States, January 2019–September 2020. *MMWR Morb Mortal Wkly Rep.* 2020;69:1841-1867. doi:10.15585/mmwr.mm6949a1

3. Lee SJ, Ward KP, Lee JY, Rodriguez CM. Parental social isolation and child maltreatment risk during the Covid-19 pandemic. *J Fam Violence.* 2022;37(5):813-824. doi:10.1007/s10896-020-00244-3

4. van der Kolk B. Developmental trauma disorder: toward a rational diagnosis for children with complex trauma histories. *Psychiatr Ann.* 2005;35(5):401-408. doi:10.3928/00485713-20050501-06

5. Dvir Y, Ford JD, Hill M, Frazier JA. Childhood maltreatment, emotional dysregulation, and psychiatric comorbidities. *Harv Rev Psychiatry.* 2014;22(3):149-161. doi:10.1097/HRP.0000000000000014

6. Spinazzola J, van der Kolk B, Ford JD. Developmental trauma disorder: a legacy of attachment trauma in victimized children. *J Trauma Stress.* 2021;34(4):711-720. doi:10.1002/jts.22697

7. Bowlby J. Attachment. In: Bowlby J. *Attachment and Loss.* 2nd ed. Basic Books; 1982.

8. Ainsworth MDS, Blehar MC, Waters E, Wall S. *Patterns of Attachment: A Psychological Study of the Strange Situation.* Lawrence Erlbaum Associates; 1978.

9. Pickreign Stronach E, Toth SL, Rogosch F, Oshri A, Manly JT, Cicchetti D. Child maltreatment, attachment security, and internal representations of mother and mother-child relationships. *Child Maltreat.* 2011;16(2):137-145. doi:10.1177/1077559511398294

10. Cyr C, Euser EM, Bakermans-Kranenburg MJ, Van Ijzendoorn MH. Attachment security and disorganization in maltreating and high-risk families: a series of meta-analyses. *Dev Psychopathol.* 2010;22(1):87-108. doi:10.1017/S0954579409990289

11. Godbout N, Daspe MÈ, Runtz M, Cyr G, Briere J. Childhood maltreatment, attachment, and borderline personality–related symptoms: gender-specific structural equation models. *Psychol Trauma Theory Res Pract Policy.* 2019;11(1):90-98. doi:10.1037/tra0000403

12. Simkiss DE, MacCallum F, Fan EE, Oates JM, Kimani PK, Stewart-Brown S. Validation of the mothers object relations scales in 2–4 year old children and

comparison with the child–parent relationship scale. *Health Qual Life Outcomes.* 2013;11(1):49. doi:10.1186/1477-7525-11-49

13. Pianta RC. Child-parent relationship scale. Unpublished Measure, University of Virginia. 1992.

14. Abidin RR. *Parenting stress index.* 3rd ed. Psychological Assessment Resources; 1995.

15. Kudielka BM, Kirschbaum C. Biological bases of the stress response. In: *Stress and Addiction.* Academic Press; 2007:3-19.

16. Young-Southward G, Svelnys C, Gajwani R, Bosquet Enlow M, Minnis H. Child maltreatment, autonomic nervous system responsivity, and psychopathology: current state of the literature and future directions. *Child Maltreat.* 2020;25(1):3-19. doi:10.1177/1077559519848497

17. Schär S, Mürner-Lavanchy I, Schmidt SJ, Koenig J, Kaess M. Child maltreatment and hypothalamic-pituitary-adrenal axis functioning: a systematic review and meta-analysis. *Front Neuroendocrinol.* 2022;66:100987. doi:10.1016/j.yfrne.2022.100987

18. Bernard K, Frost A, Bennett CB, Lindhiem O. Maltreatment and diurnal cortisol regulation: a meta-analysis. *Pyschoneuroendocr.* 2017;78:57-67. doi:10.1016/j.psyneuen.2017.01.005

19. Bernard K, Zwerling J, Dozier M. Effects of early adversity on young children's diurnal cortisol rhythms and externalizing behavior: cortisol and externalizing behavior. *Dev Psychobiol.* 2015;57(8):935-947. doi:10.1002/dev.21324

20. Wang Z, Li W, Cui N, et al. The association between child maltreatment and sleep disturbances among preschoolers. *Child Abuse Negl.* 2022;127:105525. doi:10.1016/j.chiabu.2022.105525

21. Saridjan NS, Kocevska D, Luijk MPCM, Jaddoe VWV, Verhulst FC, Tiemeier H. The prospective association of the diurnal cortisol rhythm with sleep duration and perceived sleeping problems in preschoolers: the generation r study. *Psychosom Med.* 2017;79(5):557-564. doi:10.1097/PSY.0000000000000440

22. Naughton AM, Maguire SA, Mann MK, et al. Emotional, behavioral, and developmental features indicative of neglect or emotional abuse in preschool children: a systematic review. *JAMA Pediatr.* 2013;167(8):769. doi:10.1001/jamapediatrics.2013.192

23. Eisenberg N, Spinrad TL, Eggum ND. Emotion-related self-regulation and its relation to children's maladjustment. *Annu Rev Clin Psychol.* 2010;6(1):495-525. doi:10.1146/annurev.clinpsy.121208.131208

24. Boldt LJ, Goffin KC, Kochanska G. The significance of early parent-child attachment for emerging regulation: a longitudinal investigation of processes and mechanisms from toddler age to preadolescence. *Dev Psychol.* 2020;56(3):431. doi:10.1037/dev0000862

25. Wolfe DA. Risk factors for child abuse perpetration. In: White JW, Koss MP, Kazdin AE, eds. *Violence Against Women and Children. Mapping the Terrain.* Volume 1. American Psychological Association; 2011:31-53.

26. Okado Y, Haskett ME. Three-year trajectories of parenting behaviors among physically abusive parents and their link to child adjustment. *Child Youth Care Forum.* 2015;44:613-633. doi:10.1007/s10566-014-9295-5

27. Speidel R, Wang L, Cummings EM, Valentino K. Longitudinal pathways of family influence on child self-regulation: the roles of parenting, family

expressiveness, and maternal sensitive guidance in the context of child maltreatment. *Dev Psychol.* 2020;56(3):608-622. doi:10.1037/dev0000782

28. Cicchetti D, Ng R. Emotional development in maltreated children. In: *Children and Emotion.* Karger Publishers; 2014:29-41.

29. Harms MB, Leitzke BT, Pollak SD. Maltreatment and emotional development. In: *Handbook of Emotional Development.* Springer. 2019:767-786.

30. Font SA, Berger LM. Child maltreatment and children's developmental trajectories in early to middle childhood. *Child Dev.* 2015;86(2):536-556. doi:10.1111/cdev.12322

31. Green MJ, Tzoumakis S, McIntyre B, et al. Childhood maltreatment and early developmental vulnerabilities at age 5 years. *Child Dev.* 2018;89(5):1599-1612. doi:10.1111/cdev.12928

32. Briggs-Gowan MJ, Carter AS, Irwin JR, Wachtel K, Cicchetti DV. The brief infant-toddler social and emotional assessment: screening for social-emotional problems and delays in competence. *J Pediatr Psychol.* 2004;29(2):143-155. doi:10.1093/jpepsy/jsh017

33. Achenbach, TM. *The Achenbach System of Empirically Based Assessment (ASEBA): Development, Findings, Theory, and Applications.* University of Vermont Research Center for Children, Youth and Families; 2009.

34. Reynolds CR, Kamphaus RW. Behavior assessment system for children: third edition. Pearson Assessments. 2015. https://www.pearsonassessments.com/store/usassessments/en/Store/Professional-Assessments/Behavior/Comprehensive/Behavior-Assessment-System-for-Children-%7C-Third-Edition-/p/100001402.html

35. Masson M, Bussieres E, East-Richard C, R-Mercier A, Cellard C. Neuropsychological profile of children, adolescents and adults experiencing maltreatment: a meta-analysis. *Clin Neuropsychol.* 2015;29(5):573-594. doi:10.1080/13854046.2015.1061057

36. Kavanaugh BC, Dupont-Frechette JA, Jerskey BA, Holler KA. Neurocognitive deficits in children and adolescents following maltreatment: neurodevelopmental consequences and neuropsychological implications of traumatic stress. *Appl Neuropsychol Child.* 2016; 6(1):64-78. doi:10.1080/21622965.2015.1079712

37. Viezel KD, Freer BD, Lowell A, Castillo JA. Cognitive abilities of maltreated children. *Psychol Sch.* 2015;52(1):92-106. doi:10.1002/pits.21809

38. Gazzaniga M, Ivry R, Mangun G. *Cognitive Neuroscience: The Biology of the Mind.* 5th ed. WW Norton & Company; 2019.

39. Cowan N. Working memory underpins cognitive development, learning and education. *Educ Psychol Rev.* 2014;26(2):197-223. doi:10.1007/s10648-013-9246-y

40. Fay-Stammbach T, Hawes DJ, Meredith P. Child maltreatment and emotional socialization associations with executive function in the preschool years. *Child Abuse Negl.* 2017;64:1-12. doi:10.1016/j.chiabu.2016.12.004

41. Demeusy EM, Handley ED, Rogosch FA, Cicchetti D, Toth SL. Early neglect and the development of aggression in toddlerhood: the role of working memory. *Child Maltreat.* 2018;23(4):344-354. doi:10.1177/1077559518778814

42. Fay-Stammbach T, Hawes DJ. Caregiver ratings and performance-based indices of executive function among preschoolers with and without maltreatment

experience. *Child Neuropsychol.* 2019;25(6):721-741. doi:10.1080/09297049.2 018.1530344

43. Cowell R, Cicchetti D, Rogosch FA, Toth SL. Child maltreatment and its effect on neurocognitive functioning: timing and chronicity matter. *Dev Psychopathol.* 2015;27(2):521-533. doi:10.1017/S0954579415000139

44. Viezel KD, Lowell A, Davis AS, Castillo J. Differential profiles of adaptive behavior of maltreated children. *Pychol Trauma Theory Reseaerch Practice Policy.* 2014;6(5):574-579. doi:10.1037/a0036718

45. Becker-Weidman A. Effects of early maltreatment on development: a descriptive study using the Vineland Adaptive Behavior Scales-II. *Child Welfare.* 2009;88:137-161.

46. Wechsler D. WPPSI: Wechsler Preschool and Primary Scales of Intelligence. 2012. https://www.pearsonassessments.com/store/usassessments/en/Store/Professional-Assessments/Cognition-%26-Neuro/Gifted-%26-Talented/Wechsler-Preschool-and-Primary-Scale-of-Intelligence-%7C-Fourth-Edition/p/100000102.html

47. Roid G, Pomplum M. The Stanford-Binet intelligence scales. In: *Contemporary Intellectual Assessment: Theories, Tests, and Issues.* 5th ed. Guilford Press; 2012: 249-268.

48. Matthews RN, Davis JL. The NEPSY-II. In: Flanagan DP, McDonough EM, eds. *Contemporary Intellectual Assessment: Theories, Tests, and Issues.* The Guilford Press; 2018:553-566.

49. Gioia G, Espy K, Isquith P. Behavior Rating Inventory of Executive Function-Preschool Version (BRIEF-P). Psychological Assessment Resources; 2003. https://www.parinc.com/Products/Pkey/26

50. Conners C. Conners Kiddie Continuous Performance Test. Multi-Health Systems; 2006. https://storefront.mhs.com/collections/conners-k-cpt-2

51. Sparrow SS, Saulnier CA, Cicchetti DV, Doll EA. Vineland Adaptive Behavior Scales, 3rd ed.: Manual. Pearson Assessments. 2016. https://www.pearsonassessments.com/store/usassessments/en/Store/Professional-Assessments/Behavior/Adaptive/Vineland-Adaptive-Behavior-Scales-%7C-Third-Edition/p/100001622.html

52. Silberg J. Assessing dissociative processes. In: *The Child Survivor - Healing Developmental Trauma and Dissociation.* 2nd ed. Routledge; 2021:47-68.

53. Cicchetti D, Banny A. A developmental psychopathology perspective on child maltreatment. In: Lewis M, Rudolph K, eds. *Handbook of Developmental Psychopathology.* Springer; 2014. doi:10.1007/978-1-4614-9608-3_37

54. Chui C, Tollenaar MS, Yang C, Elzinga BM, Zhang T, Ho HL. The loss of the self in memory: self-referential memory, childhood relational trauma, and dissociation. *Clin Psychol Sci.* 2018;7(2):265-282. doi:10.1177/ 2167702618804794

55. Putnam F, Helmers K, Trickett PK. Development, reliability, and validity of a child dissociation scale. *Child Abuse Negl.* 1993;17:731-741. doi:10.1016/s0145-2134(08)80004-x

56. Briere J, Johnson K, Bissada A, et al. The trauma symptom checklist for young children (TSCYC): reliability and association with abuse exposures in a multi-site study. *Child Abuse Negl.* 2001;25(8):1001-1014. doi:10.1016/s0145-2134 (01)00253-8

57. Bronsard G, Alessandrini M, Fond G, et al. The prevalence of mental disorders among children and adolescents in the child welfare system: a systematic review

and meta-analysis. *Medicine (Baltimore)*. 2016;95(7):e2622. doi:10.1097/MD.0000000000002622

58. Chandan JS, Thomas T, Gokhale KM, Bandyopadhyay S, Taylor J, Niranthara-kumar K. The burden of mental ill health associated with childhood maltreatment in the UK, using the Health Improvement Network database: a population-based retrospective cohort study. *Lancet Psychiatry*. 2019;6(11):926-934. doi:10.1016/S2215-0366(19)30369-4

59. Zeanah CH, Gleason M. Annual research review: attachment disorders in early childhood-clinical presentation, causes, correlates, and treatment. *J Child Psychol Psychiatry*. 2015;56(3):207-222. doi:10.1111/jcpp.12347

60. Haugaard J, Hazan C. Recognizing and treating uncommon behavioral and emotional disorders in children and adolescents who have been severely maltreated: reactive attachment disorder. *Child Maltreat*. 2004;9(2):154-160. doi:10.1177/1077559504264316

61. DC:0-5: diagnostic classification of mental health and development disorders of infancy and early childhood. Zero to Three: National Center for Clinical Infant Programs. August 2, 2017. https://www.zerotothree.org/resource/dc0-5-a-briefing-paper-on-diagnostic-classification-of-mental-health-and-developmental-disorders-of-infancy-and-early-childhood/

62. Alisic E, Zalta AK, van Wesel F, et al. Rates of post-traumatic stress disorder in trauma-exposed children and adolescents: meta-analysis. *Br J Psychiatry*. 2014;204(5):335-340. doi:10.1192/bjp.bp.113.131227

63. Scheeringa MS, Haslett N. The reliability and criterion validity of the diagnostic infant and preschool assessment: a new diagnostic instrument for young children. *Child Psychiatry Hum Dev*. 2010;41(3):299-312. doi:10.1007/s10578-009-0169-2

64. McKinnon A, Scheeringa MS, Meiser-Stedman R, Watson P, De Young A, Dalgleish T. The dimensionality of proposed DSM-5 PTSD symptoms in trauma-exposed young children. *J Abnorm Child Psychol*. 2019;47(11):1799-1809. doi:10.1007/s10802-019-00561-2

65. Choi KR, McCreary M, Ford JD, Rahmanian Koushkaki S, Kenan KN, Zima BT. Validation of the traumatic events screening inventory for ACES. *Pediatrics*. 2019;43(4). doi:10.1542/peds.2018-2546

66. Treatments and Practices. The National Child Traumatic Stress Network. Accessed July 21, 2022. https://www.nctsn.org/treatments-and-practices

67. Scheeringa MS. The diagnostic infant preschool assessment-likert version: preparation, concurrent construct validation, and test–retest reliability. *J Child Adolesc Psychopharmacol*. 2020;30(5):326-334. doi:10.1089/cap.2019.0168

Multidisciplinary Strategies for Assessment and Intervention

Tami L. Jakubowski, DNP, CPNP-PC, CSN

Objectives

After reading this chapter, the reader will be able to:

1. *Discuss the evolution and current status of child maltreatment policies in the United States.*

2. *Describe the role of school employees in recognizing child maltreatment.*

3. *Recognize the physical, behavioral, and psychological characteristics that may be present in a child experiencing maltreatment.*

Background and Significance

Children spend a large amount of time at school, providing a unique opportunity for teachers, administrators, school nurses, and other school personnel to establish positive relationships. The consistent presence of a school nurse establishes a unique opportunity to foster an ongoing relationship with children in school.[1] School nurses should be aware that students who are frequently absent or noncompliant with medical regimens may be at risk for child maltreatment.[2] Repetitive visits to the school nurse for nonspecific problems often occurs prior to children disclosing maltreatment.[3] School employees should not only encourage children to disclose if they are experiencing a problem by being friendly and open to conversation, but should also be observant of physical and behavioral clues among children. It is important for adults who regularly interact with children in school to have knowledge about possible physical, psychological, and behavioral signs of child maltreatment.

Child maltreatment has been recognized as an ongoing problem in the United States since the 1960s and was initially identified as socially unacceptable with the publication of an article by American pediatrician Henry Kempe on "The Battered Child Syndrome."[4] Over a decade later, in 1974, the United States established a national system for reporting the maltreatment of children with the Child Abuse Prevention and Treatment Act (CAPTA), which defines child maltreatment as "Any recent act or failure to act on the part of a parent or caretaker which results in death, serious physical or emotional harm, sexual abuse or exploitation, or an act or failure to act which presents an imminent risk of serious harm."[5] According to the Child Welfare Information Gateway, forms of child maltreatment include multiple forms of abuse (eg, physical, sexual, and psychological) as well as neglect and sex trafficking.[5] The National Association of School Nurses' (NASN's) position statement on the Role of the School Nurse in Prevention and Treatment of Child Maltreatment identifies that "prevention, early identification, intervention, and care of child maltreatment are critical to the physical/emotional wellbeing and academic success of students."[1]

School nurses, specifically, are viewed as serving a critical role in both assessment and recognition of early signs of child maltreatment as well as in educating the school community on how to best protect children.[1]

POLICY

By 1967, every American state had established a system requiring the report of suspected child maltreatment.[6] CAPTA approved funding to enhance each individual state's management of child maltreatment and established mandated reporter laws, which varied between states.[7] The establishment of stricter reporting laws increased case reports, and providing education to the public about child abuse and neglect became a focus during the 1980s.[7] Social supports to families were increased during the 1990s and continued to remain a focus through the next decade, focusing on prevention to decrease child maltreatment.[7] Multiple amendments to CAPTA during the 2000s continued the funding of child maltreatment prevention programs.[7] In 2003, the Center for the Study of Social Policy (CSSP) recognized 5 protective factors that promoted child and family wellbeing, which are as follows: resilience of parents, social relationships, providing needed support, knowledge of normal child development and parenting skills, and socio-emotional development in children.[8]

By 2005, the Office on Child Abuse and Neglect (OCAN) recognized the importance of protective factors by including them in their Prevention Resource Guide. An additional protective factor was added by OCAN in 2007, when the Children's Bureau recognized the importance of attachment and nurturing for children.[7] The acknowledgement of the importance of early relationships led to additional amendments to CAPTA in 2010 for the prevention and treatment of child maltreatment, including treatment programs for substance abuse, assistance for domestic violence victims, and resources for homeless children. Child maltreatment protective factors continued to be evaluated in 2012 and advised policy and programs for populations served by The Children's Bureau, which is managed by the Administration on Children, Youth, and Families (ACYF). Programs encompassed infants and children maltreated or at risk of maltreatment, children in foster care, enduring domestic violence, homeless or runaways, and pregnant and parenting teens.[7] Ten protective factors against child maltreatment were identified as a result of this review: self-regulation, relational skills, problem solving skills, involvement in positive activities, parenting competencies, caring adults, positive peers, positive community, positive school environments, and economic opportunities.[9] Since then, the focus of preventing child maltreatment has continued to be community-based, increasing childhood protective factors and implementing social services to decrease risk.[7] The 2021/22 Prevention Resource Guide concentrated on eliminating risks of child maltreatment by promoting healthy families and providing needed resources.[10]

THE SCHOOL NURSE'S ROLE

School nurses are in a unique position to provide interprofessional education to other professionals who routinely interact with children at school. It is imperative that school nurses educate themselves on the signs and symptoms that children may present with due to child maltreatment. School nurses also need to be aware of their state's reporting requirements for suspected child maltreatment, know how to report, and understand the manner in which reports are handled. By being informed themselves, school nurses and health room aides can provide needed education within the school setting and support when there is a suspicion of child maltreatment.

School nurses also need to support interventions aimed at developing programs to prevent child maltreatment. They can participate in the collection and analysis of data, research, and development of evidence-based practices to decrease abuse.[8] Nurses should also educate parents about normal growth and development, as well as positive parenting techniques. School nurses and teachers can benefit greatly from ongoing education in recognizing the signs of child maltreatment in order to be updated resources for the school community and allies for their students. Schools should foster the provision of trauma-informed care (TIC), a practice that is aware of the signs and symptoms of trauma, acknowledges its impact, and intervenes as necessary.[11]

PHYSICAL SIGNS OF MALTREATMENT

The most evident signs of possible child maltreatment are physical. Any child who has injuries that are unexplained such as bruises, burns, bites, or fractures may be a victim of physical abuse. Some children, when questioned, will share that the injury was caused by a caregiver or parent.[12] Bruises are an easily visible sign of maltreatment, and it is important to note the location and pattern of bruising to help identify whether maltreatment is a possible cause.[13,14] Bruises that appear symmetrical or have well-defined borders are especially concerning.[13] When a child presents with bruising, professionals need to be aware of the developmental level of the child, inquire about what happened, and determine how likely the event described could have led to the bruise.[15] The child's medical history, ethnicity, and presence of benign hyperpigmented areas also need to be taken into consideration to ensure that bruises are not due to a medical condition.[15]

Children who are impacted by a burn injury should also be asked about the origin of the burn. Burns that involve a large body area, have clearly defined margins, or are symmetrical are suspicious for maltreatment. Scald injuries lacking evidence of hot water splashing as well as burns involving the hands, feet, buttocks, or genitals are also concerning. Children with a burn injury that crosses joints and lack burn injury in areas of flexion are unlikely to be accidental, as are grouped burn lesions and cigarette burns.[13] In addition, any child who has been absent from school and then returns with marks on their skin may be a victim of physical abuse.[12]

PSYCHOLOGICAL SIGNS OF MALTREATMENT

Children may complain of frequent somatic complaints due to child maltreatment.[1] Teachers should pay attention to patterns of complaints from children such as they have a headache, stomachache, or are dizzy and are requesting to go to the nurse. Some children will show signs of depression or suicidal thoughts in response to maltreatment.[16]

BEHAVIORAL SIGNS OF MALTREATMENT

Children who develop sudden changes in behavior or performance in school, including eating and sleeping habits, may be suffering from child maltreatment.[12] Younger children may appear scared of their caregiver and delay or protest leaving for home and often lack adult supervision. Some children will come to school or extracurricular activities early and leave late as an avoidance tactic since they do not want to be at home. Children may appear overly compliant in most situations but be cautious when answering questions. They may also show signs of hypervigilance. Other children may appear anxious, depressed, withdrawn, or aggressive. Children may also demonstrate challenges with learning or concentration that are not due to a diagnosed condition.[12]

SIGNS OF NEGLECT

Children who are victims of neglect may have frequent school absences. Required immunizations and medical care may be lacking. They may have poor hygiene and body odor and have inadequate clothing for the weather. Children experiencing neglect will often either take or ask others for food or money. If questioned directly, children may admit that they are responsible for themselves most of the time and lack parental supervision. Adolescents experiencing neglect are at risk for abusing drugs or alcohol.[17] Professionals can best assess for neglect by asking the child to describe what their day at home is like including details about their meals, playtime, presence of others at home, and heat/electricity/water access.[18]

School professionals should suspect possible neglect when the child's parent or care-giver exhibits an attitude of indifference to the child or appears depressed. Adults behaving irrationally or abusing alcohol or drugs are also suspect for neglect.[18]

SIGNS OF SEXUAL ABUSE

Children who suddenly refuse to attend school are concerning for sexual abuse. Children may appear to experience difficulty sitting or walking and may have bruising, bleeding, or swelling in their genital area. New onset of bedwetting or nightmares may also be a sign. A child with sexual knowledge or behavior too advanced for their age may be a victim of sexual abuse. Children younger than 14 years who test positive for a sexually transmitted infection or pregnancy require further investigation. Most certainly, children who report sexual abuse require notification of law enforcement and pediatric emergency care for child maltreatment.[19,20]

SIGNS OF EMOTIONAL MALTREATMENT

Children who demonstrate behavioral extremes, such as aggressive or challenging behavior or extreme submissiveness, should raise concern for emotional maltreatment. Some children will act younger than their chronological age, while others will demonstrate adult-like behaviors such as supervising younger children as a parent would.[16]

Parental behaviors can also be "red flags" for emotional maltreatment. The parent or caregiver who displays a pattern of negative interactions with their child, including blaming, belittling, or outwardly rejecting the child, is cause for concern.[16]

CONCERNING SIGNS: PARENTS

There are multiple "red flag" behaviors that may be observed in parents that are a concern for child maltreatment. A delay in seeking medical care for a child's injury should raise questions as to why care was not sought. In addition, a parent who is unable to explain what happened to injure their child or presents conflicting explanations should be questioned further.[16,21] Parents whose story is not consistent with the child's injury or who lack concern for their child should be suspect.[16] Risk factors for child maltreatment include high stress levels with inadequate social support, a large number of children in the family, and a parent with a mental health disorder.[21]

CASE STUDIES

Case Study 9-1

Rosanna, a 6-year-old Hispanic female, was a first-grade student. The teacher noticed Rosanna itching her leg and asked if she needed to go to the school nurse. The nurse asked Rosanna what brought her in, and she quietly pointed to her leg. The nurse looked and noted 8 well-defined circumferential dark marks in a cluster. The lesions were about the diameter of a pencil eraser. When questioned about what happened, the child was silent.

Discussion

The nurse's knowledge about skin lesions that resemble a common object and are occurring in a group alerted her to the concern about physical abuse. The nurse used play to try to encourage the child to disclose what happened. She then reached out to the parents and asked what their knowledge of the lesions were, and she documented who was spoken to, their response, and the date and time of occurrence provided. The parents did not provide much information, so the nurse followed their legal responsibility to report the incidence, as the nurse suspected that the lesions were due to abuse. The state's system of mandatory reporting had to be followed. The nurse opted to not explain this mandate to the parents in order to keep the child safe.

Case Study 9-2

John, a 9-year-old male, was a frequent visitor to the nurse's office. On one occasion, he went to the office complaining of back pain. The nurse asked him to lift his shirt so she could check his back and noted multiple red elongated areas crossing his back. The nurse asked John what happened, and he said he slid into base playing baseball at recess. The nurse noted that the appearance of the marks on John's back were not consistent with the abrasion-type lesion that may be seen with the type of sports injury that John described. The lesions were in various stages of healing. After performing an examination, the nurse asked to check the rest of John's skin for similar marks and whether there was pain at any other location.

Discussion

The nurse talked with John again about the marks. She told him that the marks do not appear to be from a baseball sliding injury and asked if someone did this to him. He disclosed that it was his father who had hit him, and the nurse then assured John that he did the right thing in telling her the truth and conveyed that his safety was her main concern. She then asked about what object was used; John did not disclose anymore information. Law enforcement was then notified in addition to filing a suspected child abuse report. The nurse recommended that John go see his normal doctor for treatment and evaluation for the abuse.

Case Study 9-3

Taylor, a 12-year-old female, arrived at the nurse's office complaining of the frequent need to urinate. Taylor reluctantly answered questions regarding her symptoms and stated that she "doesn't want to talk about what happened" before the onset of her symptoms. Taylor became quiet when asked about what happened and if someone did anything to her.

Discussion

Taylor's case was especially difficult to evaluate. The nurse tried to talk with her further in order to obtain more information regarding what happened in an attempt to determine if there was a valid concern for sexual abuse, but Taylor's symptoms require further medical evaluation. Since she was a minor, a call to her parents would be indicated, expressing the need for medical follow-up. The nurse also reached out to the pediatric provider and alerted them to the possibility of a concern for abuse. At that point in time, further follow-up was in the hands of the pediatric provider. The nurse followed up with the provider as well as the child, parent, and child's teacher.

KEY POINTS

1. The recognition and interventions related to child maltreatment have evolved over the past 60 years.

2. Children experiencing child maltreatment are at increased risk of health complications in adulthood.

3. School employees are in a unique position to recognize possible maltreatment and intervene on behalf of children.

REFERENCES

1. Freeland M, Easterling T, Reiner K, Amidon C. Prevention and treatment of child maltreatment: the role of the school nurse. National Association of School Nurses. June 2018.

2. Welch Holmes B, Sheetz A, Allison M, et al. Role of the school nurse in providing school health services. *Pediatrics.* 2016;121(5):1052-1056. doi:10.1542/peds.2008-0382

3. Thomas R. School nurses and CSE: keep on looking and listening. *Br J School Nurs.* 2018;13(3):150-151. doi:10.12968/bjsn.2018.13.3.150

4. Kempe CH, Silverman FN, Steele BR, Droegemueller W, Silver HK. The battered-child syndrome. *JAMA.* 1962;181(1):17-24. doi:10.1001/jama.1962.03050270019004

5. Child Maltreatment 2016. US Department of Health and Human Services. 2018. Accessed June 20, 2022. https://www.acf.hhs.gov/cb/report/child-maltreatment-2016

6. The child abuse prevention and treatment act: 40 years of safeguarding America's children. National Child Abuse and Neglect Training and Publications Project. 2014. Accessed June 20, 2022. https://www.acf.hhs.gov/sites/default/files/cb/capta_40yrs.pdf

7. Child maltreatment prevention: past, present, and future. US Department of Health and Human Services, Children's Bureau. 2017. Accessed June 15, 2022. https://www.childwelfare.gov/resources/child-maltreatment-prevention-past-present-and-future/

8. Harper Browne C. The strengthening families approach and protective factors framework: branching out and reaching deeper. Center for the Study of Social Policy. 2014. Accessed June 30, 2022. https://cssp.org/resource/the-strengthening-families-approach-and-protective-factors-framework-branching-out-and-reaching-deeper/

9. Promoting protective factors for in-risk families and youth: a guide for practitioners. US Department of Health and Human Services, Children's Bureau. 2015. Accessed July 5, 2022. https://www.childwelfare.gov/pubPDFs/in_risk.pdf

10. US Department of Health and Human Services, Administration for Children and Families, Administration on Children, Youth and Families, Children's Bureau. 2021/2022 prevention resource guide. Accessed June 20, 2022. https://preventchildabuse.org/wp-content/uploads/2021/04/prevention-resource-guide-2021.pdf

11. Adverse childhood experiences study (ACE). Centers for Disease Control and Prevention. 2010. www.cdc.gov/ace/index.htm

12. What is child abuse and neglect? Recognizing the signs and symptoms. Child Welfare Information Gateway. 2019. Accessed July 9, 2022. https://www.childwelfare.gov/pubPDFs/whatiscan.pdf

13. Lucas C, Crowell K, Olympia R. Red flags and red herrings: improving the recognition of bruises and burns associated with physical abuse in school-age children. *NASN Sch Nurse.* 2021;36(1):32-38. doi:10.1177/1942602X20942922

14. Petska HW, Frasier LD, Livingston N, Moles R, Sheets LK. Patterned bruises from abusive squeezing. *Pediatr Emerg Care.* 2021;37(6):351-353. doi:10.1097/PEC.0000000000001717

15. Makaroff KL, McGraw ML. Skin conditions confused with child abuse. In: Jenny C, ed. *Child Abuse and Neglect: Diagnosis, Treatment, and Evidence.* Elsevier Saunders; 2011:252-259.

16. Fact sheet: emotional child abuse. Prevent Child Abuse America. 2016. http://www.preventchildabuse.org/images/docs/emotionalchildabuse.pdf

17. Tracy N. Signs of child neglect and how to report neglect. Healthy Place. 2018. Accessed on July 10, 2022. https://www.healthyplace.com/abuse/child-abuse-information/signs-of-child-neglect-and-how-to-report-child-neglect

18. Tracy N. What is child neglect? Healthy Place. 2018. Accessed on July 10, 2022. https://www.healthyplace.com/abuse/child-abuse-information/what-is-child-neglect

19. Sexual abuse. American Academy of Adolescent Psychology. 2014. Accessed on July 10, 2022. https://www.aacap.org/AACAP/Families_and_Youth/Facts_for_Families/FFF-Guide?Child-Sexual-Abuse-009.aspx

20. Child sexual abuse. RAINN. 2018. Accessed on July 10, 2022. https://rainn.org/articles/child-sexual-abuse

21. Pittner K, Bekermans-Kranenburg M, Alink Lenneke R, et al. Estimating the heritability of experiencing child maltreatment in an extended family design. *Child Maltreat.* 2020;35(3):289-99. doi:10.1177/10775595198888587

ADOLESCENTS WHO COMMIT SEXUAL OFFENSES

Sara Jones, PhD, APRN, PMHNP-BC, FAAN, FAANP

OBJECTIVES

After reading this chapter, the reader will be able to:

1. Identify the differences between adolescents who commit sexual offenses and adults who sexually offend.

2. Analyze the theoretical etiologies of sexual offending behaviors in adolescents.

3. Describe 4 assessment tools that can be used to help assess the risk of recidivism among adolescents who commit sexual offenses.

BACKGROUND AND SIGNIFICANCE

Between 2016 and 2020, there was an average of 225 000 sexual assaults reported in the United States.[1] It is estimated that juveniles are responsible for at least 1/4 of sexual offenses in the United States and Canada.[2,3] In addition, they account for 1/2 of all sexual offenses perpetrated against those younger than 18 years.[4] Adolescents who sexually offend (ASOs) are "[those] between the ages of 12 and 18 who have been charged with or convicted of a sexual crime, or have engaged in an act that could officially be charged as a sexual crime, or have committed any sexual act with a person of any age in an aggressive, threatening, or exploitative manner."[5] However, ASOs encompass more than this simple definition. First, they are not simply miniature versions of adult sex offenders.[6] The majority of ASOs do not go on to sexually offend during adulthood, nor are they likely to meet criteria for "pedophilia" as designated by the *Diagnostic and Statistical Manual of Mental Disorders* (DSM-5).[4,7] In regard to recidivism, ASOs sexually recidivate at lower rates than adult sex offenders.[4] Instead, they are much more likely to non-sexually reoffend, although they have less extensive criminal histories compared to their non-sex offending peers.[8] Because of these differences, the judicial system and clinicians are implementing new policies and programs to manage and prevent future adolescent sexual offending. This chapter will address issues relevant to clinical practice regarding ASOs, including theories of etiology, a system of classification, and risk assessment tools.

ETIOLOGY THEORIES

Understanding the etiologies of sexual offending can be useful in guiding the assessment and treatment of individuals who sexually offend. Many factors have been considered as an explanation for adult sexual offending, such as poor social skills, fear of rejection, anger toward women, low self-esteem, feelings of personal inadequacy, personal history of sexual victimization, exposure to violence, and atypical sexual interests.[8] Many of these factors have been implied to also play a role in adolescent sexual offending; however, research has shown that ASOs are not homogenous to adult offenders, even in their etiologies. Studies have speculated the various etiologies for years. In 2010, a meta-analysis of 59 independent studies compared male ASOs with male adolescent non-sexual offenders.[8] Eight main theories were supported by these studies and are further discussed below. It is important to remember that, although these theories provide empirical evidence to explain sexual offending, no single theory is all-inclusive. Even among existing theories there are overlaps, which demonstrates the importance of completing a thorough clinical assessment of each ASO to best guide treatment.

GENERAL DELINQUENCY

"General delinquency" is one of the proposed theories that is used to distinguish ASOs. Factors associated with general delinquency include antisocial personality traits, pro-criminal attitudes and beliefs, conduct problems, substance abuse, and association with delinquent peers.[8] These factors have been found to contribute to both sexual and non-sexual offending in adolescents. They have also been found to be risk factors for recidivism.[9] Still, one study has shown that general delinquency is significantly lower in ASOs compared to non-sexually offending adolescents, particularly in regard to recidivism.[10] Although many ASOs have a history of multiple non-sexual offenses, the sexual offense tends to be the inciting incident to a long trajectory of criminal history. When re-offending occurs, the crimes thereafter are more likely to be non-sexual in nature.[8] Hence, it is particularly uncommon to see adolescents who commit crimes that are only sexually offensive.

THE SEXUALLY ABUSED SEXUAL ABUSER

The "sexually abused sexual abuser" theory suggests that children who are sexually abused are at a higher risk to commit sexual offenses after having been a victim themselves.[8] Not all ASOs have been sexually abused, but overall, rates of sexual victimization histories are higher in ASOs than in the general population.[11] When comparing ASOs to adolescent non-sex offenders, ASOs report being sexually abused 5 times more than non-sex offenders.[8] Factors that contribute to the likelihood of a sexually abused adolescent sexually offending include whether the abuse was perpetrated by both men and women, if the perpetrator was a relative, the amount of force used, the length of time the abuse continued, and if the acts included penetration. Those who are most likely to offend experienced abuse at a younger age by both male and female relatives for long periods of time.[12] Most commonly, these adolescents mimic their own abuse when offending. Their relationship to their victim will be the same as that with their perpetrator, the means of coercion or force will be similar, and the acts themselves are most often identical.[13]

SOCIAL LEARNING THEORY

"Social learning theory" is one approach used to link personal sexual victimization to adolescent sexual offending.[12,13] As discussed above, ASOs tend to sexually offend using the same modus operandi as their perpetrator. Social learning theory suggests that an offender's first offense is committed due to an internal belief that sexual offending is acceptable.[13] Also, as a victim, the adolescent offender has a preconceived anticipation of gratification related to offending due to what they perceive their own offender obtaining. These factors create a cognitive distortion about what appropriate sexual behaviors are and alter perceptions of potential victims. Social learning theory asserts that adolescents continue to offend due to a need to resolve their own trauma related to sexual abuse. Repeat offenses may also be associated with a conditioned response related to personal sexual gratification or to release anxiety caused by the conflict of offending.

POOR CHILDHOOD ATTACHMENT

"Poor childhood attachment" is a concept used to explain a plethora of problems in adults and adolescents alike. The concept extends back to Bowlby's attachment theory,[14] which suggests that child and caregiver interactions, or the lack thereof, directly affect adult psychopathology. It is hypothesized that insecure parent-child attachment can lead to limited skills for developing appropriate intimate relationships.[15] For adolescents, little or no attachment can impact self-awareness and emotion regulation, as well as abilities to empathize for and be intimate with others.[14] In combination, these factors fuel attempts to fulfill intimacy needs using a more coercive interpersonal style. If sexual acts fulfill the adolescent's need for intimacy, recidivism is more likely to occur. Conversely, studies also suggest that strong attachments and bonds during childhood can reduce the risk of recidivism.[16]

SOCIAL INCOMPETENCE

Expanding on the above etiology, the "social incompetence" theory suggests that ASOs are not able to form appropriate and consensual relationships.[8] In fact, known risk factors for adolescent sexual offending are limited intellectual and social capacities, as well as poor social networks.[17] When adolescents have difficulty approaching and engaging with others due to these factors, they may choose to interact with individuals who they can more easily coerce, such as much younger children or vulnerable peers. These relationships are then used to fulfill their emotional and sexual needs. When evaluating the role of social incompetency in sexual offending, studies have repeatedly found that ASOs score significantly lower on both performance measures of and self-reporting about their abilities to socially interact with others, especially with peers of the opposite sex.[8] ASOs have also specifically demonstrated more social isolation compared to other adolescents, including non-sexual offenders.

ATYPICAL SEXUAL INTERESTS

A primary distinguishing factor between ASOs and other adolescents is the higher prevalence of reported atypical sexual interests.[5] Compared to their non-sexually offending peers, ASOs report more sexual deviance and more rape fantasies.[18] They also report less trust in their personal abilities to have sexual relationships with peers their own age, which may explain sexually assaulting younger individuals and the use of force or coercion. The use of pornography seems not to differ between ASOs and non-offending peers, but legal troubles as a result of pornography use (eg, underage pornography, sharing pornography without consent) is higher among ASOs.[18] When viewing depictions of children or acts of coercive sex with peers, ASOs have been confirmed to have the same physiological response of arousal and gratification as adult sex offenders.

Atypical sexual interests are significant risk factors for recidivism.[5] Still, it is important to recognize that sexual interests and arousals in adolescents are dynamic, and due to their changing nature, they should not be considered solid predictors or targets of treatment for ASOs.

PSYCHOPATHOLOGY

A recurring theory related to ASOs focuses on the direct role of psychopathology. Psychiatric disturbances, such as anxiety disorders, major depression, and personality disorders, are prevalent diagnoses found in ASOs.[8] Many of these diagnoses are biologically linked to disturbances in levels of neurotransmitters in the brain system.[19] Such neurotransmitters, including serotonin and norepinephrine, are not only associated with mood and aggressive behavior, but also with sexual behavior.[20] Still, questions of this causality arise when the psychopathology theory is analyzed (eg, are there biological or environmental conditions that precede the psychopathology?). As previous theories have suggested, ASOs may have altered childhood experiences, such as a history of sexual victimization or poor caregiver attachment, and these incidences contribute to the psychopathologies used to explain sexual offending.[11] In contrast, ASOs also report high levels of anxiety and depressive symptoms related to committing a sexual offense. In the case of psychopathology, the continuum of which came first may not be clear.

COGNITIVE ABILITIES

While individuals with impaired cognitive and intellectual abilities are overrepresented in the legal system, these traits are especially seen in those who commit sexual offenses.[17,21] Primary distinguishing factors among ASOs compared to non-sex offending peers are learning problems and other disabilities.[8] Stemming back to the theory of social incompetence, cognitive impairments can also cause an individual to be rejected by peers, which can lead to inappropriate relationships with children or coercive relationships with peers. In addition, ASOs with intellectual disabilities (compared to those without) show impaired moral reasoning, in that, they seem to justify the acts based on ideals of reciprocity. Either way, persons with impaired cognitive abilities often have poorer impulse control and lack appropriate judgment, which can pose risk factors for sexual offending.

CLASSIFICATION OF ADOLESCENTS WHO SEXUALLY OFFEND

Providers knowing the type of offender that they are treating is crucial. In the past, treatment programs for ASOs have been modeled after adult treatment programs with the assumption that sexual offending is a lifelong pattern of behaviors. Similarly, the criteria used to classify ASOs have been adopted from adult models. However, research has repeatedly shown the differences between adult sex offenders and ASOs, and, as a result, specific classification criteria for adolescents have been developed. There are various means of classifying ASOs, but current evidence best supports classifying ASOs by victim age, dividing them into adolescents who offend against children, adolescents who offend against peers or adults, and adolescents who offend against both children and adults.[22] There is also recent evidence to support consideration of offender-victim age difference when considering this classification.[23]

ADOLESCENTS WHO OFFEND AGAINST CHILDREN

Studies have shown a significant clinical difference between adolescents who offend against children versus peers or adults.[22] The definition of offenders against children varies slightly in the literature. Some literature defines offenders against children whose victims are 4 years of age or less, while other literature defines the victims to be between 3 to 12 years of age.[22,24] Compared to those who offend against peers or adults, offenders against children are typically more familiar with the victim, more likely to be related, and younger at the age of their first offense.[22] They are more likely to be males and are less likely to use force or weapons. They are also less likely to be under the influence of drugs or alcohol when offending. Developmentally, they typically demonstrate more social dysfunction and psychosocial problems. Offenders against children tend to lack confidence and fear ridicule and rejection by their peers. They view themselves as socially inadequate and overall are pessimistic about life. In addition, symptoms of depression and anxiety are more prevalent in ASOs who offend against children. One study has shown that this group is also more likely to have experienced their own traumas early in life, particularly sexual abuse.[23]

ADOLESCENTS WHO OFFEND AGAINST PEERS OR ADULTS

Adolescents who offend against peers or adults tend to have more than 1 victim, while those who offend against children typically have a single victim that they repeatedly assault.[24] Males in this category almost exclusively offend against female victims who are acquaintances, where those who offend against children are less discriminate and more likely to offend against males who are related to them. Offenders against peers/adults have less psychosocial disturbances, demonstrate more general delinquencies, and have more age-appropriate, consensual sex. They use more force and coercion, and are more likely to offend with little or no planning.[24] Their cognitive abilities are typically normal to high, and their parents/caregivers have more trouble providing help and support.[23] Lastly, they consistently exhibit a lower level of sexual preoccupation when compared to offenders against children who exhibit higher levels of deviant sexual arousal. Characteristics of adolescents who offend against peers or adults correlate with a higher prevalence of exposure to domestic abuse toward women and community violence.

THE MIXED-TYPE OFFENDER

A mixed-type offending ASO, by definition, has 2 or more victims that are diverse in age. Similar to peer/adult offenders, they are more likely to report experiences of age-appropriate consensual sex, as well as use of traditional pornography, compared to child offenders.[24] Unique to this group is that they report more atypical/deviant sexual interests and fantasies. They are likely to begin offending earlier than both child and peer/adult offenders. They also offend against both males and females, as well as both relatives and strangers. Overall, mixed-type offenders are indiscriminate when choosing their victims. Additionally, mixed-type offenders have a much greater history of non-sexual offenses compared to the other types of offenders. They have greater deficits related to affective disorders, including lack of remorse, empathy, and responsibility. Due to the varying nature of this type, evidence shows that mixed-type offenders benefit the least from treatment,[24] which indicates a higher risk of recidivism for this type.

RISK ASSESSMENTS

When assessing ASOs, both clinicians and the legal system consider a risk assessment to evaluate the risk of recidivism[25] and to provide effective treatment.[26] The purpose of this assessment is to guide the development of individual treatment plans and the level of intervention(s) needed, determine the level of supervision required to monitor the adolescent, and properly inform others involved in the risk management process. As of the publication of this book, there are multiple tools available to assess individuals' personal characteristics, histories, and behaviors, as well as the existence of present problems and the likelihood that the problems will reoccur. These tools need to be comprehensive and elastic enough to address each factor that theoretically may contribute to reoffending. The most prevalently used tools are the Juvenile Sex Offender Assessment Protocol II (J-SOAP II), the Estimate of Risk of Adolescent Sex Offender Recidivism (ERASOR), the Juvenile Sexual Offense Recidivism Risk Assessment Tool-II (JSORRAT II), the Multiple Empirically Guided Inventory of Ecological Aggregates for Assessing Sexually Abusive Adolescents and Children (MEGA), and, more recently, the Structured Assessment of Violence Risk in Youth (SAVRY). It is important to remember, however, that there are no empirically validated resources to classify long-term risk of ASOs.[27] Each tool addresses different variables along a continuum of behaviors that may contribute to reoffending. The overall goal is to accurately assess the risk of recidivism of ASOs on a scale of offenses that are less severe to those who have seriously and dangerously offended. Many assessors find that there is not a singular tool that provides an accurate assessment; current best practice is to use multiple tools in combination. It is under the discretion of individual assessors to decide which tools provide the most accurate risk assessment for each adolescent, and although formal risk assessments are helpful, they should be used in conjunction with other assessment tools and clinical judgment.

J-SOAP II

The J-SOAP was originally developed in 1998, after systematically reviewing literature related to ASOs.[27] It was revised in 2000 and again in 2003, creating the J-SOAP II. The purpose of the J-SOAP II is to predict the risk of sexual and non-sexual recidivism among males aged 12 to 18 years. It is administered by a trained clinician and can be used with adolescents who have sexually offended, as well as those with sexually coercive behaviors. It consists of 28 items indictive of risk factors for recidivism, grouped into 4 subscales: Sexual Drive/Preoccupation scale (8 items), Impulsive/Antisocial scale (8 items), Intervention scale (7 items), and

Community Stability/Adjustment scale (5 items). The first two scales assess dynamic risk factors, which are factors that can change over time, while the latter two address static risk factors, which are factors that will never change.[27,28] The Community Stability/Adjustment scale is omitted for those incarcerated or in residential treatment. Overall scores are numerical, but cutoff scores that predict risk are not indicated.[27]

ERASOR

The ERASOR was first developed in 2000 and revised in 2001 (creating Version 2.0) with the intention to be used to structure clinical interviews with ASOs ages 12 to 18.[28] Using the ERASOR, the clinician is prompted to inquire about empirically known risk factors and, ultimately, use clinical judgment to determine results. It is intended to evaluate risk for 1 year at most and not to predict long-term risk. After 1 year, the assessment should be readministered. The developers of ERASOR considered adolescence (between the ages of 12 and 18) to be a time of rapid development in areas such as sexual, social, familial, and cognitive functioning. Consisting of 25 items,[23] it considers both dynamic risk factors (16 items) and static risk factors (9 items).[28] The dynamic factors are to be coded using a 6-month time frame and are placed into 5 scales: Sexual Interests, Attitudes, and Behaviors; Historical Sexual Assaults; Psychosocial Functioning; Family/Environmental Functioning; and Treatment.

JSORRAT II

The JSORRAT-II was developed based on an actuarial approach with the goal to limit the application of adult risk factors associated with sexual offending in ASO assessment tools.[24] It identifies 12 items, all of which are static or historical, likely to demonstrate risk of recidivism.[28] The items are categorized into 4 factors: Persistence of Offending, Antisocial Orientation (Unwillingness or Inability to Follow Rules), Abuse History/Treatment Needs, and Risk Taking.

MEGA

The MEGA assesses the levels of risk of sexual offending in all children and adolescents ages 4 to 19 years.[29] It has been used with specialty populations, including offenders with developmental and intellectual delays, female and transgender offenders, and offenders younger than 12 years. The MEGA includes calibrated risk categories based on known algorithms, such as the relationship between risk and protective factors and how they factor in according to age and gender of the ASO. Consideration can also be made based on intellectual functioning. These elements are present so that the assessment not only addresses negative risk factors, but also addresses protective factors that may counteract their risk. There are 4 scales: Risk Scale, rated low, moderate, high, and very-high; Protective scale, which identifies variables that may mitigate risk; Estrangement, which indicates ASOs' relationships and interactions within; and Historic Correlative, which considers concerns related to past sexual misconduct.[29,30] It is the responsibility of the clinician to evaluate the transactions between each aggregate, identify the factors that may be associated with sexually offending for each individual, and identify protective factors.

SAVRY

The SAVRY was not specifically developed for ASOs, but for adolescents who have committed criminal offenses.[31] Still, the relevance is clear because it was developed to encourage greater consideration of protective factors that decrease risk of recidivism of any type.[32] The objective is to let the data guide utilization of the most appropriate interventions to mitigate risk through focusing on protective factors. Again, while not its intended purpose, some studies have also shown its usefulness to assess change of risk over time.[31] The SAVRY includes 30 items and 4 factors, the first 3 of which are risk factors: Historical (10 items; ie, peer delinquency), Social (6 items; ie, relationships), and Individual (8 items; ie, anger problems). The last factor assessed is Protective (6 items).[32]

CONCLUSION

Sexual offending in adolescents is a growing area in need of attention from the health care community. The developmental tasks during adolescence are conducive to the possibility of effective interventions, noting that the issues are addressed and specialized treatment is implemented. The purpose of this chapter is to provide an introduction of adolescent sexual offending for clinicians and other professionals who work with ASOs. The information is presented with aims to prevent preconceived biases and judgments and to promote awareness of a means to help this population. Introductory terms and concepts provide a foundation for understanding, but all providers must seek out their own state's statutes to know what constitutes an offense, an offender, and a victim. While there are multiple theories and typologies that attempt to explain this concept, providers must also use their own clinical judgment to assess and identify factors specific to each individual. Risk assessment tools are helpful, but should always be used by a collaborating team of clinicians trained in this area. The knowledge base about ASOs will continue to grow as the research community is constantly adding empirical evidence to aid in the assessment, treatment, and monitoring of this population.

CASE STUDY

Case Study 10-1

Alex was a 16-year-old boy who met 14-year-old Alison at a house party thrown by a friend whose parents were out of town. Alex and Alison immediately "hit it off." In fact, they were having such a good time at the party that Alison decided to go upstairs to one of the empty bedrooms to get to know Alex better. They had a few beers, and as Alison later described, they were both feeling "buzzed." While in the bedroom and sitting on the side of the bed, Alex started to kiss Alison, and moved his hand up her skirt. When she resisted, he became belligerent, pushed her onto the floor, and told her she was a "slut" to have gone with him, because she "should have known what was going to happen." He then held her down on the floor and forced his fingers inside of her vagina while forcibly kissing her, saying "you know you want this; that's why you brought me up here." Following the sexual assault, Alex and Alison rejoined the rest of the party. Alex cooled down and offered Alison another beer as if nothing ever happened, joking and laughing with other party attendees. Alison said "no" and that she wanted to go home. Alex said this was okay but told Alison that he still wanted to see her again soon and that she was now "his girl." Alison was confused and upset. Because she was unsure that what she experienced was truly sexual assault, she waited until 3 days later to report her assault to the police.

Discussion

As is often the case with adolescents who offend against peers, Alex took advantage of this situation with little to no planning. He found himself in an isolated location with a vulnerable potential victim who was impaired from alcohol. Additionally, his own cognitive abilities were impaired with alcohol. His level of sexual preoccupation was low; rather, the act of sex was more of an act of power and control for completion than any dynamic of relational intimacy or grooming. This was further demonstrated with his subsequent commentary that he then considered Alison to be "his girl."

KEY POINTS

1. Adolescents who commit sexual offenses, when compared to adult sexual offenders, typically do not go on to sexually offend during adulthood, nor are they likely to meet criteria for pedophilia. They sexually recidivate at lower rates than adult sex offenders, are much more likely to non-sexually reoffend, and have less extensive criminal histories compared to their non-sex offending peers due to their response to treatment.

2. Adolescents who commit sexual offenses can be classified by victim age. This classification includes adolescents who offend against children, against peers or adults, and against a combination of children, peers, and adults.

3. There are no empirically validated resources to classify long-term risk of ASOs reoffending; therefore, using multiple tools is the best common practice. While

formal risk assessments are helpful, they should be used in conjunction with other assessment tools and clinical judgment.

REFERENCES

1. Morgan RE, Thompson A. Criminal victimization, 2020 – supplemental statistical tables. Bureau of Justice Statistics. February 2022. https://bjs.ojp.gov/content/pub/pdf/cv20sst.pdf

2. Cale J, Smallbone S, Rayment-McHugh S, Dowling C. Offense trajectories, the unfolding of sexual and non-sexual criminal activity, and sex offense characteristics of adolescent sex offenders. *Sex Abuse*. 2016;28(8):791-812. doi:10.1177/1079063215580968

3. Rotenberg C, Cotter A. Police-reported sexual assaults in Canada before and after #MeToo, 2016 and 2017. The Canadian Center for Justice Statistics. November 8, 2018. https://www150.statcan.gc.ca/n1/en/pub/85-002-x/2018001/article/54979-eng.pdf?st=gx71dTi-

4. Ryan EP. Juvenile sex offenders. *Child Adolesc Psychiatr Clin N Am*. 2016;25(1): 81-97. doi:10.1016/j.chc.2015.08.010

5. Ryan EP, Otonichar JM. Juvenile sex offenders. *Curr Psychiatry Rep*. 2016;18(7): 67. doi:10.1007/s11920-016-0706-1

6. Carpentier J, Proulx J. Recidivism rates of treated, non-treated and dropout adolescent who have sexually offended: a non-randomized study. *Front Psychol*. 2021;12:757242. doi:10.3389/fpsyg.2021.757242

7. American Psychological Association. *Diagnostic and Statistical Manual of Mental Disorders (DSM-5)*. 5th ed. American Psychiatric Publishing; 2013.

8. Seto MC, Lalumière ML. What is so special about male adolescent sexual offending? A review and test of explanations through meta-analysis. *Psychol Bull*. 2010;136(4):526-575. doi:10.1037/a0019700

9. Mulder E, Brand E, Bullens R, van Marle H. Risk factors for overall recidivism and severity of recidivism in serious juvenile offenders. *Int J Offender Ther Comp Criminol*. 2011;55(1):118-135. doi:10.1177/0306624x09356683

10. van der Put CE, van Vugt ES, Stams GJ, Dekovi M, van der Laan PH. Differences in the prevalence and impact of risk factors for general recidivism between different types of juveniles who have committed sexual offenses (JSOs) and juveniles who have committed nonsexual offenses (NSOs). *Sex Abuse*. 2013;25(1): 41-68. doi:10.1177/1079063212452615

11. Dillard R, Beaujolais B. Trauma and adolescents who engage in sexually abusive behavior: a review of the literature. *J Child Sex Abus*. 2019;28(6):629-648. doi: 10.1080/10538712.2019.1598528

12. Lateef R, Jenney A. Understanding sexually victimized male adolescents with sexually abusive behaviors: a narrative review and clinical implications. *Trauma Violence Abuse*. 2021;22(5):1169-1180. doi:10.1177/1524838020906558

13. Burton DL, Miller DL, Shill CT. A social learning theory comparison of the sexual victimization of adolescent sexual offenders and nonsexual offending male delinquents. *Child Abuse Negl*. 2002;26(9):893-907. doi:10.1016/s0145-2134 (02)00360-5

14. Baker E, Beech AR. Dissociation and variability of adult attachment dimensions and early maladaptive schemas in sexual and violent offenders. *J Interpers Violence*. 2004;19(10):1119-1136. doi:10.1177/0886260504269091

15. Maniglio R. The role of parent-child bonding, attachment, and interpersonal problems in the development of deviant sexual fantasies in sexual offenders. *Trauma Violence Abuse.* 2012;13(2):83-96. doi:10.1177/1524838012440337

16. Spice A, Viljoen JL, Latzman NE, Scalora MJ, Ullman D. Risk and protective factors for recidivism among juveniles who have offended sexually. *Sex Abuse.* 2013;25(4):347-369. doi:10.1177/1079063212459086

17. Mulder E, Brand E, Bullens R, Van Marle H. A classification of risk factors in serious juvenile offenders and the relation between patterns of risk factors and recidivism. *Crim Behav Ment Health.* 2010;20(1):23-38. doi:10.1002/cbm.754

18. Driemeyer W, Spehr A, Yoon D, Richter-Appelt H, Briken P. Comparing sexuality, aggressiveness, and antisocial behavior of alleged juvenile sexual and violent offenders. *J Forensic Sci.* 2013;58(3):711-718. doi:10.1111/1556-4029.12086

19. Stahl SM, Lee-Zimmerman C, Cartwright S, Morrissette DA. Serotonergic drugs for depression and beyond. *Curr Drug Targets.* 2013;14(5):578-585. doi:10.2174/1389450111314050007

20. Yanowitch R, Coccaro EF. The neurochemistry of human aggression. *Adv Genet.* 2011;75:151-169. doi:10.1016/b978-0-12-380858-5.00005-8

21. van Vugt E, Asscher J, Stams GJ, Hendriks J, Bijleveld C, van der Laan P. Moral judgment of young sex offenders with and without intellectual disabilities. *Res Dev Disabil.* 2011;32(6):2841-2846. doi:10.1016/j.ridd.2011.05.022

22. Aebi M, Vogt G, Plattner B, Steinhausen HC, Bessler C. Offender types and criminality dimensions in male juveniles convicted of sexual offenses. *Sex Abuse.* 2012;24(3):265-288. doi:10.1177/1079063211420449

23. Jensen M, Smid SC, Bøe T. Characteristics of adolescent boys who have displayed harmful sexual behaviour (HSB) against children of younger or equal age. *BMC Psychol.* 2020;8(1):121. doi:10.1186/s40359-020-00490-6

24. Lillard CM, Cooper-Lehki C, Fremouw WJ, DiSciullo VA. Differences in psychosexual development among child, peer, and mixed juvenile sex offenders. *J Forensic Sci.* 2020;65(2):526-534. doi:10.1111/1556-4029.14194

25. Hempel I, Buck N, Cima M, van Marle H. Review of risk assessment instruments for juvenile sex offenders: what is next? *Int J Offender Ther Comp Criminol.* 2013;57(2):208-228. doi:10.1177/0306624x11428315

26. Barra S, Bessler C, Landolt MA, Aebi M. Testing the validity of criminal risk assessment tools in sexually abusive youth. *Psychol Assess.* 2018;30(11):1430-1443. doi:10.1037/pas0000590

27. Viljoen JL, Mordell S, Beneteau JL. Prediction of adolescent sexual reoffending: a meta-analysis of the J-SOAP-II, ERASOR, J-SORRAT-II, and Static-99. *Law Hum Behav.* 2012;36(5):423-438. doi:10.1037/h0093938

28. Chu CM, Ng K, Fong J, Teoh J. Assessing youth who sexually offended: the predictive validity of the ERASOR, J-SOAP-II, and YLS/CMI in a non-Western context. *Sex Abuse.* 2012;24(2):153-174. doi:10.1177/1079063211404250

29. Miccio-Fonseca LC. Contemporary Risk assessment tools: should we use them for sexually abusive children ages 4 to 12 years? *J Child Adolesc Trauma.* 2020;13(2):141-151. doi:10.1007/s40653-019-00267-z

30. Miccio-Fonseca LC, Rasmussen LA. MEGA --Empirical Support for Nomenclature on the Anomalies: Sexually Violent and Predatory Youth. *Int J Offender Ther Comp Criminol.* 2015;59(11):1222-1238. doi:10.1177/0306624x14533265

31. Viljoen JL, Gray AL, Shaffer C, Latzman NE, Scalora MJ, Ullman D. Changes in J-SOAP-II and SAVRY scores over the course of residential, cognitive-behavioral treatment for adolescent sexual offending. *Sex Abuse.* 2017;29(4): 342-374. doi:10.1177/1079063215595404

32. Ortega-Campos E, García-García J, De la Fuente-Sánchez L, Zaldívar-Basurto F. Assessing the interactions between strengths and risk factors of recidivism through the Structured Assessment of Violence Risk in Youth (SAVRY). *Int J Environ Res Public Health.* 2020;17(6):2112. doi:10.3390/ijerph17062112

APPLICATION OF PSYCHOMETRICS TO CHILD MALTREATMENT ASSESSMENT INSTRUMENTS

David T. Solomon, PhD, HSP-P
Jacob R. Brown, BS

OBJECTIVES

After reading this chapter, the reader will be able to:

1. *Differentiate between the various types of reliability and validity.*

2. *Evaluate assessment tools on the basis of reliability and validity.*

3. *Understand the importance of psychometrics as they pertain to measurement of psychological constructs related to child maltreatment.*

BACKGROUND AND SIGNIFICANCE

Broadly speaking, the word "psychometrics" refers to the field of study concerned with the measurement of psychological constructs. For example, behaviors, attitudes, and symptoms are all things that can vary within and across people but often cannot be directly measured in the way that attributes such as weight, height, or age can be. However, being able to accurately measure these former constructs is important for clinical and other applied reasons. For example, when treating a maltreated child for post-traumatic stress disorder (PTSD), progress monitoring can be aided by periodically measuring PTSD severity using a given instrument; in this case, PTSD is the more intangible construct of interest, and psychometrics tell us how well it is being measured. In addition to clinical applications of psychometrics, research findings that are often used to guide clinical work could be inaccurate if the instruments used in the study are not reliable and valid (these terms are elaborated on in the sections below). Readers should note that the terms, "measures," "instruments," "inventories," "tests," and "scales" will be used interchangeably, as these are all different forms of tools that are used to measure psychological constructs relevant to child maltreatment. While there are technical differences between some of these terms, those semantic differences are beyond the scope of this chapter and have little practical significance to clinical work. This chapter also occasionally uses the term "respondent" to refer to clients, research participants, or others who fill out tests and measures.

Generally, psychometric-related discussions can be broken into 2 content areas: ***reliability of measurement*** and ***validity of measurement***. When referencing a specific instrument, these content areas are considered the measure's "psychometric properties." Together, they indicate how consistently the instrument is able to measure the construct that it is measuring (ie, its reliability), and whether it is actually measuring what it is proposing to measure (ie, its validity). As noted below, there are multiple subtypes of reliability and validity. It should be noted that there is no perfect method for creating a measure with the "best" reliability and validity, and indeed some methods may strengthen some types of reliability or validity and weaken others. While these are fundamental considerations for those who construct assessment instruments, they are also important things to consider when selecting an instrument to use in an applied setting. Further, given the high-stakes nature of some psychological assessments, clinicians should have a strong understanding of psychometrics and how to discern the psychometric properties of a given measure.

The field of psychometrics is concerned with being able to index and subsequently communicate the accuracy and effectiveness of various instruments for their given purposes. For example, this would include evaluating if an inventory meant to measure child PTSD symptoms actually measures PTSD symptoms (as opposed to measuring more generalized anxiety or distress). Furthermore, these test characteristics have meaningful clinical and ethical implications. For example, the Child Abuse Potential Inventory (CAPI) is a measure meant to predict if a parent or primary caregiver is currently engaging in physical child abuse or is likely to engage in physical child abuse in the future.[1] The CAPI is sometimes used by child welfare agencies to make important placement decisions, such as whether a child will be removed from or returned to caregiver custody. Should the CAPI be inaccurate or ineffective at predicting child abuse potential, incorrect decisions could be made, causing undue harm to children and families. Other measures may be used to aid in diagnoses and treatment selection, which is important given that many interventions are designed to target certain types of symptoms and problems.

The outcomes of child maltreatment can be numerous and range in intensity. One child who has experienced trauma may develop more PTSD-specific symptoms (eg, intrusive memories, avoidance of trauma reminders) and may therefore benefit more from a treatment such as trauma-focused cognitive behavioral therapy. Another child may respond with externalizing symptoms (eg, behavioral problems) and difficulty with attachment and thus may respond better to a treatment such as parent-child interaction therapy. Thus, valid and reliable measures may aid in making these distinctions and improving treatment planning. Finally, as stated above, clinicians may also use instruments for progress monitoring. If the instrument chosen is not reliable, it may appear that the client's symptoms are not changing when they are, or alternatively, the symptoms may be improving or worsening without the measure detecting that change (ie, scores on the measure may stay the same when symptoms are in fact changing). If the instrument is not valid, it may be measuring something other than the symptoms the clinician wishes to address, which, again, could lead a clinician to make incorrect conclusions about the effectiveness of a treatment.

RELIABILITY

Reliability is a fundamental starting point for the evaluation of an instrument's psychometric properties. As noted above, reliability is often defined as the consistency of measurement. However, it may be more accurate to describe reliability as how free from error a measurement is. Indeed, measurement reliability is threatened by error, which could be anything other than the actual presence of the attribute being measured that will impact the test-taker's score. In classical test theory, an observed score (ie, the actual score obtained on the measure) on an instrument is considered to be a combination of a true score (ie, the test-taker's actual level of whatever is being measured) and any amount of error that is impacting the true score.[2] For example, most modern intelligence tests are highly reliable, meaning the scores they yield tend to be good representations of a person's ability, thus they are an examiner's best estimate of a person's intelligence quotient (IQ) score. However, sources of error such as test-taker fatigue, the examinee guessing answers correctly, or misadministration of items by the examiner may also impact these scores. When sources of error are small and infrequent, they tend to have little impact on the observed score (eg, guessing 1 item correctly does not usually drastically increase a person's final score on a test). Sources of error may also "even out" across a test when some sources of error might artificially increase a score and other sources might artificially decrease them. Therefore, even though some error is always expected, the observed scores for well-developed tests can still be good estimates if the errors are small.

Reliability coefficients, then, are numeric representations of the degree to which the observed score represents the true level of what is being measured. Reliability (as well as validity) is often reported as a correlation coefficient (eg, Pearson's r) wherein the higher the value (with +1 being the maximum), the more reliable the score. Thus, the more error in your measurement (for any given reason), the lower your coefficient will be. Generally speaking, the reliability of an instrument's scores is considered to be acceptable when the reliability coefficient is at least 0.7.[3] Below this number, the demonstrated reliability is questionable. However, depending on the measure in question and its purpose, this rule of thumb may need to be adjusted upwardly. Instruments used in high stakes testing situations, such as those described above, are held to higher psychometric standards than other instruments. For this reason, they need to yield reliable coefficients of a greater magnitude to be considered appropriate. For example, when looking at the score of an individual in a clinical setting, reliability estimates closer to 0.9 or above may be preferred.[4]

A number of factors can impact the reliability of a measure, such as **homogeneity of item content** and the number of items on the measure. Homogeneity of item content refers to the idea that items should be similar in terms of what they are measuring. For example, 2 things that are similar should correlate with one another to a higher degree, so responses to items with similar content should correlate more highly with each other than items with dissimilar (ie, heterogeneous) content. Further, the number of items on the measure also impacts reliability to a substantial degree; more items generally yield greater reliability. It should be expected that no one item is ever going to be perfect. For example, consider a childhood maltreatment questionnaire with an item such as, "Were you physically abused as a child?" As it pertains to reliability, there are many sources of error that may impact a person's answer to this item. Some may have experienced significant verbal abuse as a child, but they do not consider that to be abuse, therefore they answer "no" to this question. Others may have experienced strict parenting that does not meet most definitions of abuse, but they themselves define it that way, and thus answer, "yes." Still others may have experienced some form of abuse when they were very young and do not remember; some may know they experienced abuse but may be unwilling to say so. This one item would therefore only be reliably measuring a history of child abuse for those who had a good understanding of the definitions of abuse (a tall order given the various types of abuse and even multiple definitions of abuse across locations and research studies), a good memory of whether or not they had experienced such abuse, and a willingness to disclose their history; all other responses are being impacted by various types of error.

Any given item on a measure is subject to many types of error, including the ones mentioned in the above example. Notice that some of the types of error are idiosyncratic to the person reading the item (eg, what they consider to be abuse). It is not possible to account for every way a respondent may interpret an item. However, when a measurement has a sufficient number of well-written items, the impact of random error impacting any single item lessens. Part of the reason for this is purely mathematical. Imagine a student is a very good speller (ie, their level of the construct of "spelling ability" is very high). The night before a spelling test, the student is extremely sick and still feels ill the next day while taking the test. As a result, they do poorly on the test, not because they are a bad speller but because of the external factors of sickness and fatigue. These are essentially sources of error that have impacted the child's observed score on the spelling test, making it lower than their true spelling ability. Further, if the student only has 2 spelling tests a semester, this 1 erroneous grade highly impacts their final grade in spelling, but if the student had 10 other spelling tests, it would have a much lower impact on their final spelling grade. Thus, their final spelling grade, which is composed of more quizzes instead of just a few, is a more reliable (lower in error) indicator of their actual spelling ability. In this example, there was nothing inherently wrong with the spelling test on the day the child was sick, but some other random error impacting the child's score was still introduced. Similarly, if there are more items on a measurement, a few "fluke" responses to some items will have less impact on the overall score.

Note that this does not mean any specific item is bad per se, as there are many idiosyncratic reasons a person may respond differently to an item or interpret an item differently than others do. Still, during the scale development process, items should be scrutinized to determine if they are difficult to understand or interpret, loaded, leading, or have other issues. Producing stronger items undoubtedly reduces error related to their interpretation. For example, a respondent may be more likely to endorse the item, "Did a caregiver ever spank you and leave a bruise or other mark?" than they would to, "Were you ever physically abused?" The latter question is more loaded, requires interpretation from the respondent as to what constitutes abuse, and may feel more stigmatizing. Additionally, once a scale has been initially developed and administered to a sample of people, the items can be examined psychometrically to determine if editing or removing them may increase reliability. For example, many data analysis software used to examine the psychometric properties of measures will indicate whether removing a specific item would lower or increase the measure's overall reliability.

Finally, clinicians using measures would be wise to not over-interpret any one of a client's responses to any singular item. For example, items similar to "I can usually tell what other people are thinking" are often found on scales of delusional disorders. While such items are endorsed more often by individuals with a delusional disorder and are highly correlated with other items measuring delusional disorders (making these items perfectly acceptable to include on such scales), clients may have idiosyncratic reasons for endorsing this item that are not related to a delusional disorder. For example, a person might feel like they are very good at reading body language, or a socially anxious client may generally believe that other people usually are judging them. However, it would be equally problematic to discard scores on a measure that has been shown to be reliable and valid because of the possibility of a few fluke responses to a few items; as stated above, these types of idiosyncratic error tend to be trivial in the presence of a sufficient number of well-performing items. Overall, total scores tend to be more informative than individual scores.

TYPES OF RELIABILITY

There are several different types of reliability. First, there is *test-retest reliability*, which is the consistency of scores from the same test-takers on the same instrument across 2 points in time. To examine test-retest reliability, for example, a researcher could give the CAPI to a group of individuals at 1 point in time, then give it again after a period of time has passed, during which the score would not be expected to change. If a person's scores are high at time 1, then they would be expected to be high at time 2, and vice versa. If this is the case, then the scores received at the 2 points in time will be highly correlated, and test-retest reliability has been supported. Of note, there are no set time intervals between the assessment administrations that have been agreed upon. It largely depends on the construct being measured, as one would need to determine how long the construct would be expected to remain stable. For example, mental health symptoms may ebb and flow over time, so a shorter test-retest interval may be more necessary for measures of mental health than for measures of more stable attributes, such as personality traits.

As an example, the Childhood Trauma Questionnaire (CTQ) is a measure used to screen adults for histories of childhood maltreatment, containing subscales (ie, smaller sets of items from the overall inventory measuring more specific facets of the construct) covering physical abuse, physical neglect, emotional abuse, emotional neglect, and sexual abuse.[5] Because the measure is meant for adults to report their childhood histories, their scores should remain stable over long periods of times because their childhood histories are set and should not change. As would be expected, the test-retest reliability scores have been found to be fairly high. One sample of outpatient substance misuse clients was administered the CTQ and then retested again between 1.6 and 5.6 months later. Test-retest reliability estimates for the 5 types of maltreatment ranged from 0.79 (for physical neglect) to 0.81 (emotional neglect and sexual abuse) and 0.86 for the overall scale totaling all the items.[5] It should be noted that the overall scale, despite having more varied items (ie, being less homogeneous), has higher reliability than any given subscale. This is again indicative that scales with more items tend to have higher reliability.

Alternate form reliability is examined when 2 or more equivalent forms of the same measure are developed, which is more common with ability or achievement tests. This type of reliability is used when individuals may need to be tested multiple times. Being tested multiple times is less of an issue for mental health, personality, or other instruments that measure a person's current feelings or thoughts. However, when being tested on abilities or skills, it is possible that the person may perform better on each subsequent testing because they are becoming acquainted with the specific items. This phenomenon is referred to as "practice effects." For this reason, some test developers develop multiple versions of the same test that cover the same content areas, but that use different questions. One issue with creating 2 versions of the same test is that it may be difficult to ensure that both versions have similar difficulty; one person taking both tests should score similarly on each. Thus, when investigating alternate form reliability, each test-taker takes both forms of the assessment, and then their scores on both versions of the test are correlated. If the test-takers score similar to their own performance on both forms, then there is evidence for alternate form reliability. Because alternate form reliability applies more to ability and achievement testing, it may seem that it is not relevant to the field of child maltreatment, though there are some situations in which it may be important. For instance, if a researcher wants to determine the impact of early child maltreatment on cognitive abilities and would like to test children multiple times over a period of months or years, it would be useful for that researcher to choose a test that has multiple versions with high alternate form reliability. Otherwise, it could appear that participants' cognitive abilities are getting better, when in reality they are staying stable or getting worse, because practice effects (a type of error in this case) has artificially increased their observed scores across time.

Inter-rater reliability is the consistency of scores across raters (ie, the people who are scoring the measurement). While most tests administered are not scored by 2 different people, it should be the case that the same responses given to 2 different raters should be scored similarly. For example, if one rater calculates a total score of 25, the other should also calculate a total score of 25. Most measures are simple to score and require no subjective judgement, as most inventories present the person completing the measure with a fixed set of options, and each option has an assigned value (eg, a participant may receive a score of 5 for every item to which they select the "strongly agree" answer choice). The person scoring the measure must simply add up the values assigned to each of the examinee's responses. Some instruments are scored automatically by computer, leaving less room for human error. Therefore, inter-rater reliability is most relevant for measures that require the person administering it to convert longer narrative responses from open-ended questions into numeric options. Inter-rater reliability tends to be higher when the criteria for scoring items is more specific and objective.

One relevant measure is the Dyadic Parent-Child Interaction Coding System 4th edition (DPICS).[6] The DPICS is a behavior rating scale in which parent verbalizations and physical behaviors towards their children are identified by a trained observer and placed into several categories such as praises, negative talk (ie, criticism), commands, questions, negative touch, positive touch, and more. The DPICS is an integral part of some treatments relevant to children who have been impacted by child maltreatment, such as parent-child interaction therapy. While it is a complex coding system, the manual provides multiple examples and detailed information on each category. For example, while there is some subjectivity in what words and phrases are positive enough to be considered praises, the DPICS manual provides a table with multiple examples of words considered sufficiently positive enough to be considered praise (eg, good, terrific) and those not considered sufficiently positive enough (eg, interesting, okay). Inter-rater reliability is often calculated using the kappa coefficient; without going into too much detail about the calculations, kappa coefficients measure the extent to which independent raters agree on categorical classifications while taking into consideration the likelihood of chance agreement. The DPICS manual reports kappa coefficients for all DPICS categories in the adequate range,[6] with another study by Shanley & Niec[7] reporting all kappa values ranging from 0.8 to 0.98, which is considered almost perfect agreement. This provides evidence that the DPICS has good inter-rater reliability, with raters successfully able to apply the DPICS criteria to reach similar ratings.

Internal consistency reliability is often the type of reliability that is reported in research reports when discussing the psychometric properties of a given instrument. The logic behind internal consistency reliability is the notion that if all items on an inventory are measuring the same thing, they should have a fairly strong correlation with one another (eg, someone with high levels of depression scores high on all items asking about depression). Thus, internal consistency reliability may be more impacted by heterogeneous item content than other types of reliability. Two types of internal consistency reliability include split-half reliability and Cronbach's alpha, the latter of which has become one of the most highly reported indicators of reliability.

Split-half reliability is a type of reliability that measures how half of the items on a measure correlate with the other half of the items. To examine this type of reliability, a researcher will administer the measure to one group of individuals. They will then calculate a score for all of the odd-numbered items for each participant and a score for all of the even-numbered items before calculating the correlation coefficient between the 2 scores derived from the halves. A high correlation coefficient is evidence of good split-half reliability.

The more common type of internal consistency reliability is expressed with what is known as ***Cronbach's alpha*** (α), which is a number that expresses how similar all of the items on a scale are to one another. This number is essentially the average correlation between each item and every other item on a measure. In other words, each item is correlated with every other item, and all of these correlations are averaged (there are some additional steps in the calculation, but this is the basic unit of the formula). Using this method, it can be determined if any individual item is making the measure less reliable, in which case those items may be removed. For this reason, internal consistency reliability is a popular choice for many measure developers, especially with the advent of computer programs that can more easily calculate this score. In some instances, items with relatively suboptimal performance in this area may be retained depending on whether they contribute meaningful information when evaluating the construct.

VALIDITY

Validity is the other side of the psychometric coin and, much like reliability, cannot be overlooked when considering the psychometric properties of an assessment tool.

While reliability is concerned with how error free a measure is, validity is concerned with whether the measure is actually reflecting the construct it is supposed to measure. Some of the same properties of reliability would also apply to validity estimates. Like reliability, many types of validity estimates are based on correlations. However, whereas reliability is often measured by how well an inventory correlates with itself (eg, test-retest reliability is the correlation between a group of respondents' scores on the same test given at two different time points), validity is often measured by correlating an inventory with other inventories or outcomes. The process of evaluating validity is usually guided by theory. Specifically, based on what they know about the construct they are trying to measure, test developers theorize how their measure should relate to other measures of similar and different constructs, and then they test those hypotheses through correlations. For this reason, unlike reliability, higher correlations are not always better, and in some cases lower correlations are expected, as is the case with discriminate validity discussed below. For example, we would expect a measure of math ability to correlate highest with another measure of math ability, slightly less high with a measure of intelligence, and lowest or not at all with a measure of sociability. As with reliability, what is a "good" or "acceptable" validity depends somewhat on the purpose of the measure. For example, making decisions related to suicide risk is high stakes, as not accurately identifying a person who is at risk may eventually result in that person attempting suicide, whereas incorrectly identifying someone who is not at risk as being at risk could result in unwarranted negative consequences such as hospitalization. Thus, a measure of suicide risk used for clinical decision making would require very high predictive validity (see below) to ethically support its use.

Much like reliability, there are a number of different types of validity.

TYPES OF VALIDITY

Content validity refers to the degree to which the measure adequately reflects the full range of content related to what is being measured. For example, if an inventory was intended to measure PTSD but only asked about re-experiencing symptoms (eg, flashbacks) it does not have good content validity, as the construct of PTSD also includes hypervigilance, avoidance, and other mood symptoms. Some methods for strengthening certain types of reliability and validity may weaken others. For example, if a construct is multifaceted, it may require many different (ie, heterogeneous) types of items to fully measure the attribute. Thus, adding a wider variety of items may increase a measure's content validity but weaken its internal consistency (recall that internal consistency estimates are higher when all the items have very similar content). In some cases, item content may be so heterogeneous that it is only appropriate to examine the internal consistency of specific subscales. For instance, imagine a researcher is developing a parenting scale for children to rate how often they perceive their caregivers are engaging in various behaviors. The researcher may want to increase content validity by adding questions on positive parenting practices, such as the use of support, as well as potentially harmful parenting practices, such as the use of harsh physical punishment. For such a measure, the overall internal consistency would be low—in fact, it would not make sense to calculate a total score—but specific subscales may show good reliability and have practical utility.

Face validity refers to the degree to which the items on a measure *look* like they are measuring what they are intended to measure at face value. For example, if a PTSD measure had an item such as, "I often eat too much," the item would seem tangential and not representative of the most common symptoms of PTSD, thus lacking face validity. However, the same item would appear to have higher face validity on a scale of unhealthy eating. Unlike the other types of validity, which are typically measured using correlation coefficients similar to most types of reliability, content and face validity are typically examined using more subjective methods, such as through evaluation of the measure using expert judges.[7] It should also be noted that high face validity could be problematic in situations where respondents may have reasons to want to present themselves in a certain way. When this occurs, if a client is easily able to guess what is being measured, they may purposefully give inaccurate responses. For example, many parents presenting for a parenting capacity evaluation would answer, "No" to an item obviously measuring child maltreatment, such as, "My child has gone without having their needs met while in my care." Because of this, some measures also include "validity scales" intended to detect purposeful misrepresentation of scores. For example, the Minnesota Multiphasic Personality Inventory (MMPI)[8] asks clients about minor personal faults that most people have and would admit to. Such items can help detect a person who is "faking good" (ie, trying to appear more moral or well-adjusted than they actually are). Alternately, the MMPI also asks about uncommon symptoms that even people with genuine difficulty are unlikely to have. These items can help detect a person who is "faking bad" (ie, trying to appear worse off than they actually are). However, validity scales are somewhat rare and may occasionally yield elevated scores for respondents who are not intentionally trying to fake good or fake bad (eg, individuals who have difficulty reading and understanding the items).

Criterion validity refers to the extent to which a measure correlates with a more direct representation of the same construct (ie, the criterion). For example, a measure of aptitude for a certain job should correlate with actual performance on that job (in which case, actual performance is the criterion). In another example, measures of a mental health diagnosis could be examined to see if they relate to whether that person is diagnosed with that condition by a mental health professional (in which case, the formal diagnosis by the mental health professional is the criterion). There are 2 types of criterion validity: ***concurrent validity*** and ***predictive validity***. The difference between concurrent and predictive validity is the point in time that the criterion is measured or observed. In concurrent validity, the criterion is observed at the same time that the score on the measure of interest is obtained. In predictive validity, the measure of the criterion is measured at some point after the score on the measure is obtained.[9] In the example of the CAPI described above, determining its predictive validity might involve administering the measure to a group of parents at one time point, and then determining if the scores accurately predicted whether the family were or were not referred to a child welfare agency for child maltreatment over a follow-up period. In this case, the referral to a child welfare agency would be the criterion.

Construct validity refers to the degree to which an instrument is able to measure what it is designed to measure. Of note, this definition is synonymous with the definition of validity in general. For this reason, construct validity subsumes all other kinds of validity (ie, when examining the construct validity of a measure, one does so by evaluating the other specific types of validity mentioned). For example, the aforementioned content and criterion validity fall under the larger umbrella of construct validity. When considering whether test items are representative of what is attempting to be measured, what is actually being considered is whether they are representative of the construct.[9] Additional types of validity that fit under construct validity are ***convergent validity*** and ***discriminant validity***. Convergent validity is a type of validity that is examined when relations between scores from 2 methods of measuring the same construct are observed.[10-12] For example, when developing the CTQ mentioned above, Bernstein & Fink[5] correlated participants' scores on the CTQ with their scores on previously developed semi-structured interviews of interpersonal trauma. Discriminant validity refers to a score obtained from a measure of interest's ability to *not* correlate with content from which it is thought to be distinct. In an example given above, an examiner would *not* expect a measure of math ability to correlate highly with scores on a sociability scale. Convergent and discriminant validity are important, because if an inventory does not highly correlate with another inventory of the same construct or correlates highly with an inventory of a much different construct, it is possible that the new inventory in question is measuring something other than the desired construct. One consideration for convergent and discriminant validity is selecting appropriate comparison measures. For example, if a new math test does not correlate highly with a previously established math test, it may be unclear which test is not adequately measuring math ability. For this reason, it is useful to choose comparison measures that have been well-established as reliable and valid to eliminate the possibility that the low correlation was caused by the comparison measure being weak.

THE RELATIONSHIP BETWEEN RELIABILITY AND VALIDITY

A common example that is used to highlight the concepts of reliability and validity, as well as their relationship with each other, is that of the dartboard and bullseye (**Figure 11-1**).[7] If one was to evaluate a person's performance at hitting the bullseye in terms of their reliability, they would want to examine how consistently their darts are hitting the same area of the board. If the examinee is hitting different places every time they throw, then they are not very reliable. However, if they usually hit the same place, or at least very close to the same place, every time, they are reliable. Notice that this example says nothing about hitting what they are aiming for on the board. Accuracy is not a requirement for reliability. One can have a reliably bad aim even if they always hit the same place on the outer portion of the board. Comparing this metaphor to psychological measurement, an instrument might be remarkably reliable at measuring depression, such that people with similar levels of depression will obtain similar scores, and the same person taking the same instrument multiple times will get the same score. However, if the instrument is intended to measure PTSD, it is reliable but not valid. It is hitting the wrong target. In order to be good at darts, one has to be able to hit the center bullseye. This is where validity comes in. The dartboard equivalent to measuring what one is intending to measure is the ability to hit the spot they are aiming for. That is, having good aim highlights the concept of being both a valid and reliable measure. However, if someone only occasionally hits the bullseye or tends to hit random places on the target, they cannot be considered to be good at darts. This demonstrates the relationship between reliability and validity. That is, that

Figure 11-1. *Reliability and Validity Bullseye Example (Credit for Image: Charles G. Mills)*

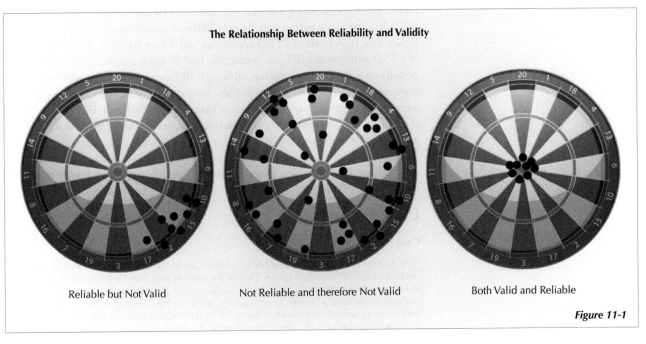

The Relationship Between Reliability and Validity

Reliable but Not Valid   Not Reliable and therefore Not Valid   Both Valid and Reliable

Figure 11-1

reliability is necessary for validity. A measure cannot be valid if it is not reliable, though, as the earlier example points out, a measure could be reliable but not valid. It is also worth noting that reliability and validity are not dichotomous concepts, as a measure's scores are not considered to be either *reliable or not reliable* or *valid or not valid*. Indeed, as discussed earlier, these concepts exist on a continuum and what is considered reliable or valid enough is often context dependent. This is not to say that there are not points at which reliability and validity coefficients are so low that the measure would not be considered for use. This is certainly the case, but that does not demonstrate an *absence* of reliability and validity; it simply demonstrates *inadequate* reliability and validity.

CONCLUSION

Assessment instruments can aid in the evaluation, treatment planning, and treatment monitoring of individuals who have experienced child maltreatment and other types of trauma. Such instruments can also aid in applied research on the reduction, prevention, and intervention of cases of childhood trauma. The psychometric properties of a given instrument are a fundamental consideration when evaluating that instrument for use in applied settings. Reliability and validity are 2 pieces of psychometric information that can help a clinician or researcher discern the degree to which a given consistent instrument measures what it is intended to measure. While every situation involving psychometric evaluation will involve nuances specific to the instrument in question, as well as the specific situation, readers should now be better equipped to subject their instruments to such considerations of their psychometric properties. This chapter focused on giving a brief, simple overview of psychometrics with particular attention given to information that would be useful to clinicians working with assessment instruments. Individuals looking for a more in-depth discussion of psychometrics (eg, those interested in developing their own tests and measures) may benefit from reviewing additional materials.

It should be noted that this chapter focused on the concepts of reliability and validity as they pertain to classical test theory, which, as mentioned above, examines the combination of sources of error with an individual's true score on some construct to yield the observed score they received. Applying this theory, assessment developers seek to reduce the sources of error to the extent possible so that the observed score is as close as it can be to the true score. A newer theory, item response theory (IRT), utilizes sophisticated computer modeling to examine the relationship between an individual's response to a given item and the level of a given construct present within the individual (eg, a person may be only likely to answer "true" to a given test item if they have high levels of PTSD symptoms, not if they have low or moderate levels of PTSD symptoms).[2] IRT can potentially lead to more precise representations of a person's true score on a construct. Although IRT can provide a number of ways to improve the reliability of a measure (eg, by accounting for the impact of random guessing), it requires a large sample size of examinees to develop an IRT measure and is more often used with computer-administered testing such as the SAT. As such, IRT is less applicable to the assessments currently relevant to child maltreatment assessment. However, recent research has begun to use IRT to develop measures related to adults who have experienced abuse, meaning that IRT may become important in this field in the future.[13]

CASE STUDY

Case Study 11-1

Amy Acevedo was a licensed psychological associate in the state of North Carolina who worked for a child advocacy center. One of the services they provided was parental capacity evaluations for families with Child Protective Services (CPS) involvement. As part of this evaluation, she used a number of techniques, including interviewing, record review, and administering several psychometric measures. In determining parental capacity to protect, she had the option of using one of two instruments: the Parenting Ability and Care Inventory

(PACI) or the Malesky-Barton Parenting Scale (MBPS). Both of these were published measures, and the publishers provided manuals for each describing the norming sample and psychometric qualities of each scale. Both scales allowed the test administrator to calculate t-scores comparing the test-taker to the "typical" parent in the norming group. Ms. Acevedo noticed from the manual that the PACI and the MBPS were similar in many aspects of their psychometrics. For example, both had high test-retest reliability and internal consistency. However, there were also some notable differences. Investigating face validity, the PACI seemed to have high face validity with items such as "I sometimes spank my child when I am frustrated with their behavior." Conversely, the MBPS had items that appeared to be more related to coping skills, such as, "When I am stressed, I try to take a moment to calm myself." However, for predictive validity, the MBPS had a much stronger relationship with future CPS reports than did the PACI.

Discussion

Both of these measures were made up as hypothetical for this case study. It is important in decision making that a helping professional is able to compare a test-taker's score to the general population (eg, to determine if they are higher or lower in child maltreatment potential than other parents in the norming sample). This was shown in this example in that both measures provide t-scores that compare the person taking the measure to the average score found in the norming sample. As stated in the chapter, high face validity may not always be desirable based on what is being measured and the purpose of the assessment. In this case, a test-taker would feel the need to disagree with items that overtly dealt with child maltreatment. In this case, the MBPS had items that were dealing more with coping skills, which is related to child maltreatment potential and could be a target of intervention (ie, when parents are low in coping skills, interventions could be aimed at increasing these skills to both reduce parental distress and the likelihood of future maltreatment). In this situation, where preventing child maltreatment is paramount, predictive validity is likely one of the most important types of validity, so the MBPS should be chosen in this case, and Ms. Acevedo should choose the MBPS. Finally, it is important to note from this case study the results of any type of measure are not considered in isolation, but are considered in relation to other sources of information, such as interviews, backgrounds, and other measures.

KEY POINTS

1. Understanding psychometrics is crucial to the ability to select appropriate measures to use in applied settings.

2. Two fundamental psychometric properties are reliability and validity.

3. Reliability and validity (and the various types of each) are intrinsically intertwined and should be considered in conjunction with one another for a comprehensive understanding of the psychometric performance of a given instrument.

REFERENCES

1. Milner JS. *The Child Abuse Potential Inventory: Manual.* 2nd ed. Psytec Corporation; 1986.

2. Cappelleri JC, Jason Lundy J, Hays RD. Overview of classical test theory and item response theory for the quantitative assessment of items in developing patient-reported outcomes measures. *Clin Ther.* 2014;36(5):648-662. doi:10.1016/j.clinthera.2014.04.006

3. Yang Y, Green SB. Coefficient alpha: a reliability coefficient for the 21st century? *J Psychoeduc Assess.* 2011;29(4):377-392. doi:10.1177/0734282911406668

4. Frost MH, Reeve BB, Liepa AM, Stauffer JW, Hays RD. What is sufficient evidence for the reliability and validity of patient-reported outcome measures? *Value Health.* 2007;10(Suppl2):S94-S105. doi:10.1111/j.1524-4733.2007.00272.x

5. Bernstein DP, Fink L. *Childhood Trauma Questionnaire: A Retrospective Self-Report.* Pearson; 1998.

6. Eyberg SM, Nelson MM, Ginn NC, Bhuiyan N, Boggs SR. *Dyadic Parent-Child Interaction Coding System (DPICS) Comprehensive Manual for Research and Training.* 4th ed. PCIT International, INC; 2013.

7. Shanley JR, Niec LN. The contribution of the Dyadic Parent-Child Interaction Coding System (DPICS) warm-up segments in assessing parent-child interactions. *Child Family Behav Ther.* 2011;33(3):248-263. doi:10.1080/07317107.2011.596009

8. Ben-Porath YS, Tellegen A. *Minnesota Multiphasic Personality Inventory-3 (MMPI-3): Manual for administration, scoring, and interpretation.* University of Minnesota Press; 2020.

9. Wallace J. *Research Methods in Psychology.* Kendall Hunt; 2012.

10. Cronbach LJ, Meehl PE. Construct validity in psychological tests. *Psychol Bull.* 1955;52(4):281-300. doi:10.1037/h0040957

11. Campbell DT, Fisk DW. Convergent and discriminant validity by the multitrait-multimethod matrix. *Psychol Bull.* 1959;56(2):81. doi:10.1037/h0046016

12. Cozby P, Bates S. *Methods in Behavioral Research.* 12th ed. McGraw-Hill; 2015.

13. Antelo E, Saldaña O, Guilera G, Rodríguez-Carballeira Á. Psychosocial difficulties in survivors of group psychological abuse: development and validation of a new measure using classical test theory and item response theory. *Psychol Viol.* 2021;11(3):286-295. doi:10.1037/vio0000307.supp (Supplemental)

SUICIDE RISK AND SCREENING

Adam D. Hicks, MA

Rachel S. Faulkenberry, BS

David M. McCord, PhD

OBJECTIVES
After reading this chapter, the reader will be able to:

1. *Differentiate between suicidal/death ideation and other risk factors associated with suicide.*

2. *Differentiate between necessary components and other risk factors that are associated with the risk of dying by suicide.*

3. *Formulate their own suicide risk assessment routine or modify a pre-existing assessment to fit their current field of practice.*

BACKGROUND AND SIGNIFICANCE

Suicide is the second leading cause of death among children and young adults between the ages of 10 and 24 in the United States.[1] Of particular concern is the significant increase in suicide rates for the 10-year-old to14-year-old age group.[2] One report, using data from 2008 to 2015, indicated that the rate of hospitalizations resulting from suicide attempts had doubled during that time, with significant increases specific to the 15 to 17 age group.[3] Please see **Figure 12-1** for a chart demonstrating the pattern of attempted suicide rates in high school students from 2011 to 2021.

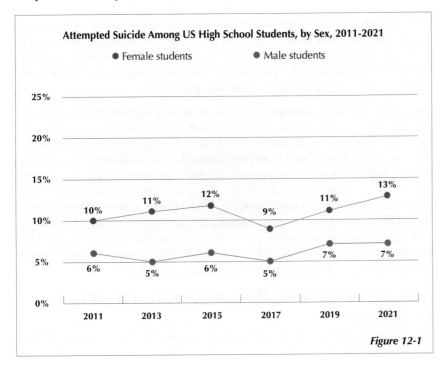

Figure 12-1. *Pattern of attempted suicides in high school students.[4]*

Attempted Suicide Among US High School Students, by Sex, 2011-2021

Figure 12-1

There is a substantial amount of literature documenting associations between childhood maltreatment and suicidal behavior during childhood, adolescence, and emerging adulthood.[5] A comprehensive meta-analysis from 2020 that focused on 79 high-quality studies, including more than 300 000 participants, yielded numerous relevant findings.[5] Suicide attempts were 3.5 times more likely when sexual abuse was present, 2 times more likely when physical abuse was present, and 2 times more likely when emotional abuse was present. Emotional and physical neglect were also associated with higher suicide rates, but did not have concrete statistics due to their inclusion in a limited number of studies.[5] Using studies that did not indicate the specific form of maltreatment, an "overall child abuse" variable was created, which was associated with 3-fold increased odds for suicide attempts.[5] Thus, it is reasonable to suggest that a history of childhood maltreatment should be formally considered as a risk factor in suicide risk assessment. Additional research has suggested that sexual abuse directly affected suicidal ideation, while emotional abuse and neglect indirectly affected suicidal ideation through dissociation and hopelessness.[6] Again, these results provide a better understanding of the links between maltreatment and suicidality, as well as direct targets for intervention.

GENERAL SIGNS OF SUICIDE RISK

Typically, the least severe sign of suicide is having thoughts about dying, which is referred to as death ideation.[7,8] Typical thoughts that fall into this category include wishing to be dead, such as wishing to "fall asleep and never wake up." Assessing for death ideation can be difficult because some patients will voice thoughts or wishes that seem to fit the profile, but upon further inquiry, their thoughts may be better categorized as being similar to cryogenic capsule concepts present in science fiction. Specifically, they may wish that they could freeze and wait until some stressful life circumstance passes or resolves. Distinguishing between death ideation and these life-pause fantasies may be complicated when working with children, especially under the age of 5, who may not have acquired the cognitive concept of death.[9]

The next step above death ideation is suicidal ideation. The distinguishing factor between these concepts is that death ideation represents a passive wish for death (eg, a religious person may say "I wish God would just take me," or more generally "I wish I were dead"), whereas suicidal ideation is more active.[7,8] When a person's desire to die increases, they tend to move from passively wishing for death to becoming the agent of their death. It is incumbent on the professional to follow up if a patient reports having thoughts about death in order to accurately differentiate between suicidal and death ideation. Some ways to clarify this with a patient would be to ask for clarification; for example, "So, you said that you were having thoughts about death. Just so I'm clear, do you ever think about killing yourself?"

Next, there are suicide attempts. A suicide attempt is different from general self-harm in that someone making a suicide attempt is acting with the knowledge and hope that their actions will lead to their death.[7,8] Leading up to a suicide attempt, the final general signs of suicide are plans, methods, and preparation. A suicide plan typically will include a set time or event that will trigger someone to attempt to kill themselves (eg, "If my partner dumps me, I'm going to try and kill myself," "If my parents divorce, I'm going to kill myself"). Methods refer to how someone plans to try to kill themselves, such as using firearms, slitting wrist/veins/arteries, overdosing, or hanging. Preparations include any steps the person has taken to prepare for a suicide attempt, including stockpiling pills, purchasing a firearm, making plans for attempting in privacy, writing a note, or giving away possessions.

THE INTERPERSONAL PSYCHOLOGICAL THEORY OF SUICIDE

The Interpersonal Psychological Theory of Suicide (IPTS) is a well-established and influential theory based on assessing the likelihood that someone will die by suicide.[7,8] The IPTS states that someone's risk of dying by suicide is associated with 2 primary factors: the desire to die and the ability to kill oneself.

THE DESIRE TO DIE

The need to belong and the need to have worth are the 2 concurrent interpersonal concerns that are related to an individual's desire to die.[7,8] These interpersonal concerns are referred to as thwarted belongingness (ie, believing that one is unwanted or has been ostracized from a social group) and perceived burdensomeness (ie, believing one is a burden to others).[9,10]

Thwarted belongingness may present in multiple ways and vary by life stage. For example, the targeted group that a person feels the need to belong to may change across their lives. Therefore, it is important for a practitioner to first ask general questions to assess if the patient feels that they are alone or unwanted.[7] If the patient reports having those feelings, then the practitioner can ask if the patient's feelings of being alone or unwanted are tied to a specific social group (eg, family, friends, clubs, sports). Perceived burdensomeness may likewise present in various ways, but is generally expressed by patients believing that their death is worth more than their life.[8] Perceived burdensomeness may be expressed as a strong sense of self-hatred and low self-worth; however, it may also be expressed with some sense of self-sacrifice (eg, "My death will help my parents because they won't have to buy things for me," "My friends will be better off with me gone because I won't pull them down [emotionally] all the time").[8] Some behavioral and demographic variables to be aware of for both thwarted belongingness and perceived burdensomeness include having few friends, being socially isolated or withdrawn, a history of child abuse or neglect, having a nonintact family, and having conflictual family relationships.[8] As such, even if a practitioner is working with an adolescent, it is important they ask about childhood maltreatment given that those experiences are associated with suicide risk in adolescents and even into adulthood.[5] Furthermore, a meta-analysis from 2017 provided evidence that both thwarted belongingness and perceived burdensomeness were associated with the development or presence of suicidal thoughts, as well as having a history of suicide attempts when a patient's ability to kill themselves was also considered.[8]

THE ABILITY TO KILL ONESELF

The ability to kill oneself is also referred to as the capability for suicide.[6] Capability for suicide stems from both inborn traits and learned behavior.[8] In terms of inborn traits, people who are more sensation-seeking may have a naturally higher capability for suicide because they often seek out experiences and are less risk averse.[8] Such individuals may engage in more dangerous behaviors that would make it easier for them to try to kill themselves if they wanted to. For example, someone who engages in street racing or reckless driving would find it easier to kill themselves by wrecking their car if they had the desire to die, than someone who is a restrictive or hesitant driver. Acquired, or learned capabilities are behaviors that someone engages in over time that will make it easier for someone to try to kill themselves. Self-harming is the most prominent example. Someone who self-harms over an extended period of time will likely raise their pain tolerance and gain a level of comfort with causing themselves pain.[6] Because the capability for suicide is independent of the desire for suicide, it is important, especially for mental health care professionals, to assess capability even if their patient denies a current desire to die.[8] Some common ways of assessing this would be to ask if there are firearms in a patient's home (if so, how are they stored), if a patient takes all medications as prescribed, and if they engage in unsafe or risky behaviors (eg, substance use, unsafe sex).

RISK OF DYING BY SUICIDE

By applying the IPTS model, one can assess a patient's level of risk of dying by suicide. The following is a quick summary of the process involved in determining a patient's level of risk (low, moderate, severe, and extreme). First, there are 3 necessary components, at least one of which must be present for a patient to be classified above low risk.[7] These necessary components include multiple previous attempts (with the most recent attempt having occurred within 2 years), current plans or preparations, and current suicidal or death ideation.[7] Apart from these necessary components, there are other risk factors that should be considered, but no specific one is necessary. These other risk factors include current or past self-harm, a family history of suicide, fearlessness about death or killing oneself, thwarted belongingness, perceived burdensomeness, hopelessness, recent stressors, and a diagnosed mental health disorder. Mood disorders, psychotic disorders, substance use disorders, impulse-control disorders, personality disorders, anxiety disorders, and eating disorders are associated with elevated risks for suicidal thoughts and death by suicide.[7]

The patient's answers to these questions will determine their level of suicide risk: Low, Moderate, Severe, and Extreme.[6] As demonstrated in **Table 12-1**, patients who have a Low risk for suicide may have 1) no necessary components or other risk factors, 2) a history of multiple attempts but have no other necessary components or risk factors, or 3) suicidal ideation, no other necessary components, and only 1 risk factor.[7] A patient would be categorized as Moderate risk if they have 1) a history of multiple attempts and one other necessary component or risk factor, 2) current plans, methods, or intent to attempt suicide but no history of attempts or other risk factors, or 3) suicidal ideation, no other necessary components, and at least 2 other risk factors.[7] A patient that meets criteria for Severe suicide risk may have 1) a history of multiple attempts and 2 other risk factors, or 2) current plans, methods, or intent to attempt suicide and 1 other risk factor.[7] Finally, a patient who meets

---

Table 12-1. Evaluating Suicide Risk

RISK LEVEL			
LOW	MODERATE	SEVERE	EXTREME
Hx of attempts – No Ideation – No Plans/prep – No Intent – NA ORF – NA	Hx of attempts – Yes (Ideation OR Plans/prep OR ORF) - Yes, <2 Intent - NA ORF – NA	Hx of attempts – Yes Ideation – NA Plans/prep – NA Intent – NA ORF – >1	Hx of attempts – Yes Ideation – NA Plans/prep – Yes Intent – Yes ORF – NA
or	or	or	or
Ideation - No Plans/prep - No Intent - NA ORF - NA	Hx of attempts – No Ideation – No (Plans/prep OR Intent) – Yes ORF – NA	Hx of attempts – NA Ideation – NA (Plans/prep OR Intent) – Yes ORF – >0	Hx of attempts – No Ideation – NA Plans/prep – Yes Intent – Yes ORF – >1
or	or		
Hx of attempts – No Ideation – Yes Plans/prep – No Intent – No ORF – <2	Hx of attempts – No Ideation – Yes Plans/prep – No Intent – No ORF – >1		

Hx of attempts = history of at least two previous attempts; Ideation = current suicidal or death ideation; Plans/prep = specific plans and preparation and method; Intent = intent to die by suicide; ORF = other risk factors; NA = item not relevant for yes/no decision regarding this specific risk category.

criteria for Extreme risk for suicide may have 1) a history of multiple attempts and current plans, methods, and intent to attempt suicide, or 2) current plans, methods, and intent to attempt suicide and 2 other risk factors with no history of multiple attempts.[7]

A patient's level of risk determines what level of intervention they require to address their suicide risk. Someone who is at a Low level of risk for suicide may still require interventions to treat other problems they may have (eg, physical health problems, mental disorders).[7] It is important to note that within the IPTS, there is not a "no risk" category; just because someone may seem to have no risk does not mean they will never develop risk.[7] In fact, suicide risk may fluctuate over short periods of time. Therefore, even for people categorized as Low risk, it is recommended that they be provided crisis or emergency help lines in case they were to need them in the future. For patients classified as Moderate risk, they should be referred to or be receiving outpatient mental health care treatment.[7] For Severe level risk, patients may require intensive outpatient treatment, whereas someone with Extreme risk will likely require inpatient hospitalization.[7] When working with children or adolescents whose parents or guardians have shown themselves to be engaged, comfortable, willing, and able, they may be able to make modifications at home, as well as increase their monitoring of their child to avoid hospitalization. Such modifications could include keeping means of suicide in secured areas (eg, firearms unloaded and stored in a gun safe, medications stored in locations inaccessible to the child or adolescent). Short-term hospitalization tends to have poor outcomes in terms of reducing someone's lifelong risk of death by suicide.[10] For more in-depth descriptions of all concepts covered here concerning the IPTS and evaluation of suicide risk, including a helpful flow-chart and table to help determine suicide risk level, please refer to Chu et al.[9]

CONSIDERATIONS SPECIFIC TO WORKING WITH CHILDREN AND ADOLESCENTS

The topic of suicide can be a difficult one to broach, no matter the situation or audience. Talking about suicide with young people is perhaps even more complicated because children experience depression and suicidality differently than adults. Knowing what to look for and what strategies are effective when dealing with young people who are at risk of dying by suicide is vital. In addition to more recognizable symptoms of depression, adolescents tend to report experiencing more physical symptoms, such as sleep difficulties or changes in appetite, which may not immediately stand out.[11] Monitoring a child and noticing when they seem to be struggling with these things can help concerned parties know when to reach out and check on the child's wellbeing and to start potentially life-saving conversations. Indications that a child is having thoughts related to suicide risk can include expressing apathy about things that used to interest them, self-loathing, or feeling hopeless or worthless.[12] These are all warning signs that children and adolescents often communicate that are important to consider in addition to explicit thoughts about wanting to die.

Some young people may feel ashamed of or uncomfortable with expressing their emotions when asked if they are struggling. Research has shown that depression and guilt can occur in children from preschool age to adolescence, and that symptom severity follows incremental patterns (eg, if a preschooler's symptoms become more severe from age 4 to age 6, then it is likely they will continue to worsen from age 6 to age 8).[13] Organizations such as the American Foundation for Suicide Prevention suggest that those providing care for children and adolescents who express thoughts related to suicide create an open and safe space for conversation. Listening to and understanding what the child is experiencing can help those concerned about their welfare to provide support and identify new potential risk factors. Starting conversations about mental health does not need to follow a specific formula but can be as simple as asking a child in plain language about their day, their feelings, or recent events in their life and keeping the conversation going from there.[14]

It is important to note that asking directly if they are experiencing thoughts about death does not increase the risk that they will die by suicide.[15] If a child is at a higher level of risk, closely monitoring symptoms, communicating directly, and addressing concerning behavior right away is imperative. Professionals can assist in managing risk and helping to secure the safety of the child.

Because child and adolescent suicide is a growing concern, proper prevention and management infrastructure is necessary to meet the needs of this population. Support can come in many forms and from a variety of sources. Family plays an incredibly important role in this context. A significant developmental and relational influence in a child's life, positive and negative familial connections can have an impact on the risk for, experience of, and treatment of adolescent suicidality.[16] Since many adolescents spend a considerable amount of time in their homes, parents are uniquely situated to build a trusting environment, facilitate communication, and intervene in their child's life when necessary. The benefits of open communication and a strong parent-child relationship extend beyond just the ability to effectively discuss depression and suicide. Better communication between adolescents and their parents is linked to more positive responses to treatment for depressed and suicidal teens.[17] Positive family involvement can also be a strong protective factor against future or continued suicidal behavior.[18] On the other hand, negative parent-child relationships not only prevent the open communication needed to address these important issues, but can also lead to an increase in factors related to suicide risk.[19] Thus, family is a particularly important consideration in child and adolescent mental health. Parents who struggle to build this relationship or want to improve communication with their child may work to build these bonds over time or seek help from a family therapist or counselor to develop the best strategies.

Primary care physicians and pediatricians are another group that can play a key role in the identification, prevention, and treatment of adolescent suicidality. One of the most effective strategies in a medical environment is widespread use of appropriate screenings for depression and suicide that can identify at-risk individuals and enable the health provider to give the best care and assistance to the patient and their family, identifying adequate safety measures where needed.[20] During a medical examination, physicians are also in a position to catch evidence of other concerning behaviors such as non-suicidal self-injury. Adolescents may resort to cutting, burning, and other forms of self-harm for many reasons, but this behavior is an indicator that a future suicide attempt is more likely and that they could be at higher risk of death by suicide.[14] Therefore, it is important that physicians take note of injuries they suspect could be self-inflicted. Primary care physicians may also intervene in more extreme cases or refer patients to more specialized treatment. Similarly, in a recent review of the topic, Pestaner et al[21] explain that school nurses are another important set of figures that are able to provide care to adolescents and children who are at Moderate risk or higher for suicide. While they are not trained physicians, they may be able to effectively recognize warning signs or troubling behaviors, refer the child to appropriate counseling or resources, and, with proper training, can conduct interventions or treatment that may assist in improving the mental health of the child.[21] Social workers often have one-on-one interactions with children and adolescents who may need additional care or suicide intervention. They can be instrumental in initiating care for these individuals and identifying their mental health needs. Another significant role they can play in the treatment and prevention of suicide is through education initiatives; they may provide resources and host workshops, trainings, or lectures for schools and communities on the dangers of suicide and methods for appropriately identifying risk among young people.[22] A more widespread understanding of the risks, warning signs, and support available can equip the community to handle this issue more effectively.

If a relative, social worker, health care provider, or other individual expresses concern that a child may be depressed or at risk of dying by suicide, then therapy or mental health counseling will likely be a beneficial next step. A trained psychologist can provide assessment and recommendations as well as support to the client and their family. For those aged 12 years and under, there has been evidence that play therapy can be adapted to help treat and prevent suicide.[23] Rather than specific forms of therapy, clinicians may provide assessment of risk and assist a parent or guardian in managing the child's safety.[24] For older children, therapy can provide a safe space to talk through feelings of depression, hopelessness, or suicidal ideation. There are many treatments available for adolescents, including Cognitive Behavioral Therapy, which is widely used to treat a range of mental health concerns, and which research suggests could function as a protective factor against suicidality.[25]

CASE STUDIES

Case Study 12-1

A 9-year-old child was brought in to see their pediatrician by their parents, who reported that their child had been staying in bed for the past 2 days saying they did not feel well. The child was not running a fever, and there were no other signs of infection or injury. The parents told the pediatrician that they knew their child had been having problems at school, but that they were having a difficult time discussing it with them.

Discussion

The pediatrician should attempt to talk to the child about their problems at school. If it seemed that the child was comfortable talking with their parents in the room, then their parents could stay; if not, the parents should be asked to step out of the room. In this case, the child reported that they were being isolated at school, had no friends, and felt alone and unwanted. The child denied having suicidal thoughts or intent to kill themselves. Because there was no evidence of imminent risk and the child was exhibiting behaviors associated with possible increases in suicide risk, the pediatrician referred the child for outpatient counseling. The pediatrician provided the parents with online resources to help them better communicate and advocate for their child.

Case Study 12-2

A 15-year-old went to their first outpatient therapy appointment. Their therapist began conducting a general intake, which included questions about suicide risk. The adolescent reported that they had experienced some thoughts about killing themselves in the past, but they said they had not been having thoughts now and that they had no intention of killing themselves.

Discussion

Even though the adolescent did not have signs of imminent risk, given this appointment was in a mental health setting, the therapist should still conduct a full risk interview. In this case, the therapist learned that the adolescent had experience hunting and handling firearms, that there were unsecured firearms in their home, and that they had little fear of death. The therapist also found out that the adolescent had a family history of suicide (an uncle) and they had been experiencing some significant stress at school. Given that this adolescent met several signs related to the ability to kill themselves and they had a past history of suicidal thoughts, the therapist should continue to monitor their risk in their future sessions.

KEY POINTS

1. There is a significant association between children and adolescents who have experienced various forms of maltreatment and their risk for suicide, which may extend into their adulthood.

2. It is important to be specific in terms of what is meant by "suicide risk," as there are many components of varying degrees that must be considered when establishing risk level.

3. Various professionals may find themselves in positions where they interact with a child or adolescent who may be at risk for suicide; though conversations about suicide are not pleasant, forming a plan for assessment can help boost your competency and confidence in doing so.

RESOURCES

— Suicide and Crisis Lifeline: 988

— American Foundation for Suicide Prevention: https://afsp.org/

— National Alliance on Mental Illness: https://www.nami.org/

— With Hope Foundation: https://www.withhopefoundation.org/

REFERENCES

1. 10 leading causes of death by age group, United States. Centers for Disease Control and Prevention. Accessed March 20, 2023. https://www.cdc.gov/injury/wisqars/pdf/leading_causes_of_death_by_age_group_2018-508.pdf

2. QuickStats: death rates for motor vehicle traffic injury, suicide, and homicide among children and adolescents aged 10–14 years — United States, 1999–2014. Centers for Disease Control and Prevention. Updated August 17, 2017. Accessed March 20, 2023. https://www.cdc.gov/mmwr/volumes/65/wr/pdfs/mm6543a8.pdf

3. Plemmons G, Hall M, Doupnik S, et al. Hospitalization for suicide ideation or attempt: 2008-2015. *Pediatrics*. 2018;141(6):e20172426. doi:10.1542/peds.2017-2426

4. Suicide and homicide death rates among youth and young adults aged 10-24: United States, 2001-2021. Centers for Disease Control and Prevention. Accessed October 4, 2023. https://www.cdc.gov/nchs/data/databriefs/db471.pdf

5. Berardelli I, Sarubbi S, Rogante E, et al. Association between childhood maltreatment and suicidal ideation: a path analysis study. *J Clin Med*. 2022;11(8):2179. doi:10.3390/jcm11082179

6. Angelakis I, Austin JL, Gooding P. Association of childhood maltreatment with suicide behaviors among young people: a systematic review and meta-analysis. *JAMA Netw Open*. 2020;3(8):e2012563. doi:10.1001/jamanetworkopen.2020.12563

7. Chu C, Klein KM, Buchman-Schmitt JM, Hom MA, Hagan CR, Joiner TE. Routinized assessment of suicide risk in clinical practice: an empirically informed update. *J Clin Psychol*. 2015;71(12):1186-200. doi:10.1002/jclp.22210

8. Chu C, Buchman-Schmitt JM, Stanley IH, et al. The interpersonal theory of suicide: a systematic review and meta-analysis of a decade of cross-national research. *Psychol Bull*. 2017;143(12):1313-1345. doi:10.1037/bul0000123

9. Talking to children about death: an age-by-age guide. Children's Hospital of Orange County. Accessed August 23, 2023. https://health.choc.org/talking-to-children-about-death-an-age-by-age-guide/

10. Chung DT, Ryan CJ, Hadzi-Pavlovic D, Singh SP, Stanton C, Large MM. Suicide rates after discharge from psychiatric facilities: a systematic review and meta-analysis. *JAMA Psychiatry*. 2017;74(7):694-702. doi:10.1001/jamapsychiatry.2017.1044

11. Rice F, Riglin L, Lomax T, et al. Adolescent and adult differences in major depression symptom profiles. *J Affect Disord*. 2019;243:175-181. doi:10.1016/j.jad.2018.09.015

12. Teens and suicide: what parents should know. American Foundation for Suicide Prevention. Accessed April 16, 2023. https://afsp.org/teens-and-suicide-what-parents-should-know/

13. Morken IS, Viddal KR, Ranum B, Wichstrom L. Depression from preschool to adolescence – five faces of stability. *J Child Psychol Psychiatry.* 2020;62:1000-1009. doi:10.1111/jcpp.13362

14. Becker M, Correll CU. Suicidality in childhood and adolescence. *Deutsches Ärzteblatt International.* 2020;117:261-267. doi:10.3238/arztebl.2020.0261

15. Valente SM. Assessing patients for suicide risk. *Nursing.* 2010;40(5)36-40. doi:10.1097/NURSE.0000371125.53758.2f

16. Frey LM, Hans JD, Sanford RL. Where is family science in suicide prevention and intervention? Theoretical applications for a systemic perspective. *J Fam Theory Rev.* 2016;8(4):446-462. doi:10.1111/jftr.12168

17. Zisk A, Abbott CH, Bounoua N, Diamond GS, Kobak R. Parent–teen communication predicts treatment benefit for depressed and suicidal adolescents. *J Consult Clin Psychol.* 2019;87(12):1137-1148. doi:10.1037/ccp0000457

18. Simões RMP, Santos JCPD, Martinho MJCM. Adolescents with suicidal behaviours: a qualitative study about the assessment of inpatient service and transition to community. *J Psychiatr Ment Health Nurs.* 2021;28(4):622-631. doi:10.1111/jpm.12707

19. Hunt QA, Ewing ESK, Weiler LM, et al. Family relationships and the interpersonal theory of suicide in a clinically suicidal sample of adolescents. *J Marital Fam Ther.* 2022;48(3):798-811. doi:10.1111/jmft.12549

20. Horowitz L, Tipton MV, Pao M. Primary and secondary prevention of youth suicide. *Pediatrics.* 2020;145(Supplement_2):S195-S203. doi:10.1542/peds.2019-2056H

21. Pestaner MC, Tyndall DE, Powell SB. The role of the school nurse in suicide interventions: an integrative review. *J Sch Nurs.*2019;37(1):41-50. doi:10.1177/1059840519889679

22. Levine J, Sher L. How to increase the role of social workers in suicide preventative interventions. *Acta Neuropsychiatr.* 2020;32(4):186-195. doi:10.1017/neu.2020.11

23. Kathryn BM, Stark C, Suri T, Brown EC. Childhood suicide: a call to action for play therapists. *Int J Play Ther.* 2023;32(4):243-257. doi:10.1037/pla0000202

24. Anderson AR, Keyes GM, Jobes DA. Understanding and treating suicidal risk in young children. *Practice Innovations.* 2020;1(1):3-19. doi:10.1037/pri0000018

25. Wolk CB, Kendall PC, Beidas RS. Cognitive-behavioral therapy for child anxiety confers long-term protection from suicidality. *J Am Acad Child Adolesc Psychiatry.* 2015;54(3):175-179. doi:10.1016/jaac.2014.12.004

Assessment

Multiple Choice

For questions 1-3, read the scenario below and answer the following questions by selecting the best response or responses from those provided.

Jane is a 13-year-old, seventh-grade child with an unremarkable medical history, including an absence of perinatal complications. Jane's academic history has largely been average. She has never been referred for special education. She currently resides with her biological mother and her mother's new boyfriend. She has started to demonstrate academic, attention, social, and emotional problems this academic year that were not previously present. Her teachers report that Jane is exhibiting increasing levels of social isolation and has largely stopped participating in class.

Jane is referred for an evaluation for Attention-Deficit/Hyperactivity Disorder (ADHD). Her mother reported the following symptoms to Jane's pediatrician: Jane does not listen to her mother when she speaks to her, does not follow directions, appears highly disorganized, will not complete activities at home that require high attention to detail (or makes careless mistakes if she is forced to do them), and is easily distracted. Using the criteria in the DSM-5, Jane is diagnosed with ADHD predominately inattentive presentation and started on methylphenidate.

1. Which of the following is the *most* likely explanation for Jane's behavior presentation?

    A. She has had ADHD for years, and it is just now manifesting

    B. Seventh grade is a difficult time for children, and these types of adjustment problems should be expected

    C. Something has changed in Jane's home environment, and the possibility of child maltreatment should be considered

    D. Jane has likely developed another psychiatric condition, such as anorexia nervosa or major depressive disorder

2. Which of the following is the *least* accurate statement if Jane is being sexually abused by her mother's boyfriend?

    A. Jane is likely to develop acute significant decline (ie, 2 standard deviation) in neurocognitive functioning, including a substantial decline in intellectual functioning

    B. Jane may develop cognitive difficulties that may not manifest for years

    C. Although Jane is not displaying sufficient symptomology to be considered for a diagnosis of major depressive disorder, she is at an increased risk of the condition as an adult

    D. Jane may display a variety of executive functioning problems, such as issues with inhibition, planning, and mental flexibility

3. Jane is now 40 years old and working as a moderately successful accountant. She never disclosed to anyone that she was sexually abused as a 13-year-old by her mother's boyfriend. Over the past few years or so, she has exhibited signs of cardiovascular disease and diabetes. Are the development of these concerns consistent with a history of childhood maltreatment?

    A. Yes

    B. No

For questions 4-6, read each question carefully and select the best response or responses from those provided.

4. What are some examples of child-level determinants that may increase the risk of maltreatment?

    A. Low neighborhood safety

    B. High family income

    C. Low birth weight

    D. Community involvement

5. How do social determinants at the community level, such as collective efficacy and social disorder, affect child maltreatment?

    A. They have no impact on child maltreatment

    B. They lead to increased positive parenting behaviors

    C. They influence parenting environments and overall community safety

    D. They only affect children's education

6. Why is it essential to recognize and address the complex dynamics between social determinants, including individual characteristics, when working to prevent child maltreatment?

    A. It is not essential, as individual characteristics do not play a role in child maltreatment

    B. Recognizing these dynamics helps in designing more effective interventions

    C. It is not essential, because child maltreatment is solely determined by parents

    D. Addressing individual characteristics causes more harm than good

For questions 7 and 8, read the scenario below and answer the following questions by selecting the best response or responses from those provided.

Caitlin was a child who aspirated feces after being left alone in a crib for 3 days as an infant. She was in the hospital for a week without predictable, warm, responsive caregivers by her side. When she was returned from the hospital, her mother abandoned her, and she was left in the care of her biological grandfather. Being physically compromised with significant health issues, he was unable to consistently care for her needs in a predictable and dependable manner. When she was 3 years old, people experienced her as avoidant, isolating, and disinterested in activities around her. She had many challenges in school and was put on punitive behavior programs that were meant to curb her violent outbursts. She was eventually expelled from kindergarten for aggression against other children when they came near her. After her grandfather passed away, she was placed in several foster placements and was unable to secure a permanent placement. When questioned, workers would say, "That's just the way she's always been."

7. How might knowing Caitlin's early beginnings influence the actions of the people in her life?

    A. It does not make a difference; she is who she is

    B. These facts highlight the gaps in her early development relationally

    C. This information can help us design consequences for her bad behavior

    D. It leads us to care for this child who has been hurt and abandoned since her early beginnings and gain the capacity to offer her comfort and hang in there for what it takes for her to heal and grow

8. How might a biographical timeline session help team members see themselves as having the capacity to be social therapists with respect to Caitlin?

    A. Team members would have the opportunity to learn from a facilitator about the developmental consequences of traumatic beginnings on Caitlin's brain, body, and behavioral patterns. They realize that events, even in the distant past, are relevant today

    B. Through the learning opportunity of the biographical timeline, the social therapists are able to reframe their previous negative feelings about Caitlin to meet their now deeper understanding of her in context to her life experiences

    C. Now that the overt behaviors have a context, a deeper understanding of a healing pathway emerges. The social therapists now feel called on to use their own skills, talents, and creativity to meet the needs of this child for whom they now have compassion

    D. All of the above

For question 9, read the scenario below and answer the following question by selecting the best response or responses from those provided.

Jordan is a 16-year-old female who was referred to your office for a clinical interview following suspected child physical abuse. School personnel reported the family to child protective services after Jordan showed up at school with bruises on her arms and torso. In your office, she sits with her arms crossed and avoids your attempts to make eye contact. Her knee rapidly bounces up and down. She tells you that she does not know why she is here and that "nothing happened." She politely responds to your questions but denies any experience of abuse before you even broach the subject in any of your questions.

9. What might be the most appropriate next step to take with Jordan?

    A. Conclude the interview, since she denies experiencing any abuse

    B. Remind her of the possible consequences of lying or withholding information

    C. Engage her in more neutral topics to build rapport and help her feel more comfortable

    D. Bring in your supervisor to see if Jordan will provide different answers when someone in a position of authority is present

For questions 10 and 11, read the scenario below and answer the following questions by selecting the best response or responses from those provided.

Arturo, an 11-year-old Hispanic boy, presents for a clinical interview after witnessing his cousin get shot outside of their home. The cousin died in the street as Arturo watched the paramedics try to save his life. As you introduce yourself, you ask him about his expectations for the interview. He responds that he knows he will need to talk about what he saw, how his cousin died, and how he has been feeling. He seems sad but willing to talk about what happened.

10. *True or False?* In your clinical interview with Arturo, you should solely focus on the identified traumatic event of his cousin's homicide that resulted in the referral.

    A. True

    B. False

11. Which of the following topics will *not* be specifically assessed during your interview with Arturo?

    A. Trauma symptoms

    B. Veracity of Arturo's statements

    C. Additional symptoms (eg, depression, anxiety, substance use)

    D. Arturo's coping skills

For questions 12-14, read the following scenario and answer the questions by selecting the best response or responses from those provided.

A school nurse is bandaging the knee of a child, Sarah, who has skinned her knee during recess. While treating the wound, the nurse notices several bruises at various levels of healing on Sarah's legs.

12. Which of these is *not* an especially concerning sign that Sarah's bruises may be the result of child maltreatment?

    A. The bruises being symmetrical

    B. The bruises having well-defined borders

    C. The bruises having appeared after Sarah has been absent from school

    D. All of the above are concerning signs

13. Which of the following are additional signs that Sarah may be experiencing maltreatment?

    A. Sarah reporting that she does not like school

    B. Sarah choosing to read during recess

    C. Sarah having little appetite during lunch when she previously ate well

    D. All of the above are additional signs

14. If the nurse suspects Sarah's bruises are the result of maltreatment, she should:

    A. Call the police

    B. Call child protective services

    C. Call the local reporting hotline

    D. Perform a full investigation and take no action until she is certain it was maltreatment

    E. Follow local mandatory reporting guidelines

For questions 15-17, read the following scenario and answer the questions by selecting the best response or responses from those provided.

Tommy is 13 years old and was recently brought in for investigation after his 6-year-old sister disclosed that he has been "making me touch his privates." During questioning, Tommy tells law enforcement, "My cousin used to do it to me, so I was just teaching my sister." As the investigation continues, it appears that Tommy's sister is his only victim. Prior to going to court, Tommy undergoes a comprehensive evaluation to assess his risk of sexually re-offending again. Since this is his only known offense, the mental health provider wants to be sure to assess not only his risk factors, but also the protective factors that may counteract the risks.

15. This scenario represents which of the following etiologies of adolescent sexual offending?

    A. General Delinquency

    B. Atypical Sexual Interests

    C. Sexually Abused Sexual Abuser

    D. Psychopathology

16. Since it appears that Tommy's sister is his only victim, which type of offender would he be classified as?

    A. Adolescent who offends against children

    B. Pedophile

    C. Adolescent who offends against peers

    D. Mixed-type offender

17. Prior to going to court, Tommy undergoes a comprehensive evaluation to assess his risk of sexually re-offending. Since this is his only known offense, the mental health provider wants to be sure to assess not only his risk factors, but also the protective factors that may counteract the risks. Which of the following assessment tools was designed for this purpose?

    A. Juvenile Sex Offender Assessment Protocol II (J-SOAP II)

    B. Estimate of Risk of Adolescent Sex Offender Recidivism (ERASOR)

    C. Juvenile Sexual Offense Recidivism Risk Assessment Tool-II (JSORRAT II)

    D. The Multiple Empirically Guided Inventory of Ecological Aggregates for Assessing Sexually Abusive Adolescents and Children (MEGA)

For questions 18-20, read the following scenario and answer the questions by selecting the best response or responses from those provided.

Dr. Chambers works at a child advocacy center that provides assessment and therapy services for children and adolescents who have experienced child maltreatment. The child advocacy center also engages in research activities with clients when appropriate consent and assent has been obtained. She wants to develop a new inventory to measure adolescent PTSD symptoms. After developing a series of items, she wants to examine the reliability and validity of her new scale.

18. When clients initially come in for services, they have 2 sessions of assessment to help determine any relevant diagnoses or symptoms prior to returning for a feedback session where the results are shared with the adolescent and their family and treatment recommendations are made. Each of these 3 sessions occur about a week apart. As a first step in examining the psychometrics of her new inventory, Dr. Chambers administers the items to 30 clients during their first intake visit, and then administers the items again to those same 30 clients at their feedback session. She then correlates the clients' responses at the first visit with their responses at the feedback session. This would be to examine:

   A. Test-retest reliability

   B. Split-half reliability

   C. Alternate form reliability

   D. Predictive validity

19. Later, Dr. Chambers examines if scores on her inventory administered during the first intake day are related to whether or not the client receives a formal diagnosis of PTSD from a licensed clinician based on a clinical interview conducted during that same intake day. She expects higher scores on her inventory will be related to a higher likelihood a client will receive a PTSD diagnosis. This would be to examine:

   A. Test-retest reliability

   B. Predictive validity

   C. Concurrent validity

   D. Discriminant validity

20. After examining the reliability and validity of her new inventory, which of the following conclusions could Dr. Chambers *not* make:

   A. Her measure is reliable, but seems to be measuring something other than PTSD, so it is not valid

   B. Her measure is not reliable, but does seem to be a valid measure of PTSD symptoms

   C. Her measure is not really reliable nor is it valid

   D. She could come to any of the above conclusions depending on the evidence

CONSTRUCTED RESPONSE

For questions 21-23, read the scenario provided and use it to formulate a response.

N is a 10-year-old, nonbinary, Caucasian child who was sexually abused by their stepfather between the ages of 7 and 9 years old. N's teacher made a report to child protective services when they disclosed information about the abuse. Since the report was made, N's mother has separated from the stepfather, who no longer lives in their house. During the initial intake session, N's mother shared that N has stopped talking to their friends, is struggling to focus in school, spends most of their time alone in their room, engages in self-harming behaviors, and has angry outbursts whenever they are asked to spend time with family or do their chores.

21. Has N experienced a single incident trauma or developmental trauma?

22. Do these concerns fit into the 3 symptom domains of Developmental Trauma Disorder?

23. What type of intervention(s) could be beneficial to N?

For questions 24 and 25, read each question carefully and provide a response.

24. What are some examples of child-level determinants that may increase the risk of maltreatment?

25. *(For this question, please refer to Caitlin's scenario, used for questions 7 and 8)* How might the knowledge of the events in Caitlin's past influence her day-to-day treatment?

For questions 26-28, read the scenario provided and use it to formulate a response.

Kyle was a 4-year-old Caucasian boy referred for group treatment by a school social worker who was concerned about a number of behavioral problems. From infancy, Kyle experienced multiple forms of maltreatment, such as witnessing his mother perpetrate psychological and physical violence toward his grandmother. Kyle was threatened with physical abuse by his mother and witnessed her substance abuse and suicide attempt. Finally, Kyle reported that one of his mother's boyfriends had touched Kyle's genitalia.

Kyle exhibited a number of concerning behaviors across a wide set of domains. At home, Kyle's behavior was defiant and rigid. When his belongings were moved or routines disrupted, Kyle reacted with explosive displays of anger that included yelling, crying, kicking, and throwing objects. Kyle's play with siblings and peers quickly turned from playful to violent. Finally, Kyle had sleep problems, waking often, having nightmares, and refusing to sleep alone. At school, Kyle had difficulty interacting appropriately with both teachers and peers, and he had few skills for coping with negative emotions. For example, he was highly sensitive to the emotional experiences of his classmates, so that when other children became distressed or upset, Kyle became agitated or angry and paced around the room. Once when another child was crying, Kyle screamed, "Make him stop; he is trying to upset me!" Kyle often attempted to self-soothe by engaging in rigid and repetitive play. When peers were aggressive or dysregulated in the class, Kyle often appeared spaced out and confused, wandering the room with little direction and speaking to himself in baby-talk. When his mother picked him up from preschool, he was known to freeze in place, pull out his hair, and run to hide. Of greatest concern was Kyle's preoccupation with death and suicide. For example, he demanded that his teachers and classmates call him "Killer." Kyle often made suicidal gestures such as holding a kitchen knife to his throat, and once, his teachers found him with a plastic bag over his head. When the teachers inquired what he was doing, Kyle claimed that he was "making suicide" like his mother.

26. Based on the description of Kyle's case, which domains of functioning are most impaired? What clinical diagnoses would you consider for Kyle and why?

27. What are 2 reasons why differential diagnosis with preschool-age children who have experienced maltreatment can be difficult?

28. Chapter 8 discusses several different domains that are affected by early childhood maltreatment. What are some ways that these domains might overlap with and affect each other, and how might this provide support for the diagnosis of Developmental Trauma Disorder?

For questions 29 and 30, read each question carefully and provide a response.

29. Sam is a 10-year-old with whom you are working. Up until today, he would often talk to you about one of his favorite video games that he plays with his friend online. Today, he made no mention of it. You inquire, "Hey Sam, you win any big matches since we last talked?" Sam says, "No, I haven't really been playing that – I don't really care about that anymore." Would his response indicate a need to do a suicide risk assessment?

30. Sarah is a 17-year-old and you just assessed her for suicide risk. Sarah recently tried to hang herself and was found by her younger brother, who was able to get her down before she experienced a significant injury. Sarah said this is the first time she has tried to kill herself, but she said she continues to experience thoughts about killing herself every day. She said she does not have a plan right now and that she is unsure if she would try again. She noted that hanging was very painful, and it scared her once she tried. She also said she has not thought about any other ways to try and kill herself, and she denied any history of purposefully injuring herself apart from her recent hanging attempt. She said that she has few friends at school, is bullied often, and feels worthless and hopeless. Sarah's parents tell you that they are not aware of any family history of suicide and that Sarah has never received mental health care treatment before. How would you rate Sarah's level of risk of dying by suicide according to the Interpersonal Psychological Theory of Suicide rating system? Explain your process for coming to that conclusion and any suggestions you would make to Sarah and her parents in terms of intervention.

ANSWER KEY

1. C
2. A
3. A
4. C
5. C
6. B
7. B, D
8. D

9. C (This case is an example of a child who may be resistant to completing a clinical interview. The most appropriate next step would be to try and build rapport with Jordan. Often, once children feel more comfortable with the evaluator, they are more willing to participate. The evaluator would not want to prematurely terminate the interview or coerce the child into participating.)

10. B (When conducting a clinical interview in the context of child exposure to trauma, it is important to conduct a broad assessment and assess for the presence of any other trauma exposures – not just the identified traumatic event. Prematurely narrowing the focus of a clinical interview on a single identified traumatic event, even if it is the reason the child has been identified for services, risks overlooking important clinical information.)

11. B (The goal of a clinical interview is to assess a child's understanding of their experiences and symptoms, explore the possible origin of symptoms, identify risk factors, evaluate strengths and coping skills, and guide further assessment in treatment. In contrast, a forensic interview may explore the veracity of a child's statements to support investigation or prosecution efforts.)

12. D

13. C (Changes in behavior, including appetite, are signs that maltreatment may be occurring. Reading during recess and reporting to not like school are likely not signs of maltreatment unless they are changes from her previous behavior.)

14. E (Mandatory reporting guidelines include how to make reports and will vary by state [eg, is there a centralized reporting hotline or are reports made directly to local child welfare agencies?]. States may also differ in where maltreatment is reported based on who is suspected of perpetrating the maltreatment [eg, a caregiver or a non-caregiver]. It should also be noted that many jurisdictions require the reporting of any suspected child maltreatment, meaning evidence or certainty are not required.)

15. C

16. A

17. D

18. A (Giving the same clients the same items at two time points and then comparing the results would be an example of test-retest reliability. Split-half reliability would require her to only give the items to the clients one time, and then correlating the odd and even items with each other. There is no alternate form in this example, which would involve two sets of different items meant to measure the same thing, so alternate form reliability does not apply. Finally, predictive validity would involve some external criterion that she intended to predict using the items, which is not the case.)

19. C (In this example, the diagnosis of PTSD would be the criterion, indicating that this is a type of criterion validity. Because the inventory is given at roughly the same time as the criterion is ascertained, it would be an example of concurrent validity. Discriminant validity would involve making sure the inventory is not related to some construct we would not expect it to be highly related to; because we would expect scores on a PTSD measure to be related to actual PTSD diagnosis, this choice does not fit. Because reliability involves comparing a measure with itself, any answer choice with the word reliability [eg, test-retest reliability] would not fit.)

20. B (Reliability is a requirement for a measure to be valid. If a measure is not reliable, it indicates it is mostly measuring error instead of measuring a specific construct. Therefore, it cannot possibly be measuring the construct of interest.)

21. N has experienced developmental trauma (sexual abuse by a caregiver).

22. Yes: emotion and somatic dysregulation, attentional or behavioral dysregulation, and self and interpersonal dysregulation.

23. Any combination of the following: Sensory Motor Arousal Regulation Treatment (SMART), Attachment, Regulation, and Competency (ARC), Trauma-Focused Cognitive Behavioral Therapy (TF-CBT), Expressive or Play-Based Interventions.

24. Child-level determinants include factors such as low birth weight, congenital diseases, poor health and development, special needs, and contact with child welfare agencies. These child-specific factors can increase the vulnerability to maltreatment.

25. Caregivers might create a day that would meet the developmental needs of Caitlin by filling in the gaps of where wounds, issues, and missed opportunities left detrimental effects. Caregivers would rise to the occasion of being trustworthy, predictable, compassionate, soothing, and patient as they work alongside Caitlin. Caregivers would also be able to access their own creativity to energize and inspire this child using a multi-sensory approach.

26. Kyle has significant affective and behavioral dysregulation, which is evident at home with his mother and siblings, as well as at school with his teachers and peers. While he also shows some attachment problems and potential dissociative symptoms, the domains of affective and behavioral dysregulation seem to be both the most pervasive and to cause the most impairment in functioning. In terms of clinical diagnoses, PTSD with dissociative features should be considered, due to his hypervigilance, nightmares, and fears (eg, of sleeping alone). Another possible consideration would be regulatory disorder based on his difficulties sleeping, or potentially reactive attachment disorder, based on his interpersonal difficulties and his unusual behavior with his mother. Finally, depression and suicidality should also be assessed, based on his suicidal behavior and his irritability and sleep problems, which could be symptoms of depression.

27. The effects of maltreatment are typically not limited to a well-defined set of symptoms that can be attributed to a single diagnosis. Instead, maltreatment often manifests in wide-ranging impairments across multiple systems of functioning. Traditional diagnoses that focus on particular subsets of symptoms (eg, depression, anxiety) may not include all the mental health problems experienced by maltreated children. Furthermore, there might be high comorbidity between diagnoses in maltreated children, meaning that they meet criteria for multiple diagnoses at once.

28. At preschool age, children do not have many skills for self-regulation. They rely heavily on their caregivers to help them learn to control their feelings and behaviors (ie, co-regulation). Problems with attachment from maltreatment might result in a lack of co-regulation between the child and caregiver, which might then result in behavioral and emotional dysregulation problems. Maltreatment also results in problems with executive functioning, which includes inhibitory control and attention, and problems with biological stress regulation systems, both of which could result in further problems with behavioral and self-regulation. Finally, maltreatment in the preschool years is also associated with dissociation, which also contributes to rapidly fluctuating emotional states and problems with attention and memory. All of these processes can overlap to contribute to the many different types of clinical internalizing and externalizing problems that are often seen in children who experience maltreatment. The Developmental Trauma Disorder (DTD) diagnosis was created to provide parsimony by accounting for the variety of symptoms experienced by maltreated children within a single diagnosis. The introduction of the DTD diagnosis should assist with differential diagnosis because it captures diverse symptoms that all stem from maltreatment.

29. Yes. First, Sam is demonstrating apathy towards a once-loved activity. In addition, because you know that Sam played this game with his online friends, his lack of engagement may indicate that something happened within his friend group that may contribute to the development of thwarted belongingness.

30. Sarah would be at a moderate risk level. Although she recently attempted to hang herself, she has no history of other attempts, so she would not be a multiple attempter. She also denied having any plans or preparations. However, she did report current and recent suicidal thoughts. In addition, she reported the presence of hopelessness, thwarted belongingness, perceived burdensomeness, and stress associated with bullying at school. It should be suggested that Sarah enter into outpatient mental health care treatment that may include both a medical referral and a referral for therapy.